"If you believe that people have no history worth mentioning, it's easy to believe they have no humanity worth defending."

—William Loren Katz

Abandoned History Series

This book is part of the Abandoned History Series published by the Museum of disABILITY History, People Inc., and People Ink Press.

Due to a general reluctance to discuss the way those in need were treated in the past, records and memories of the institutions that served the poor, sick, and disabled are fading into the past—into the world of abandoned history.

The Museum of disABILITY History is committed to preserving the important historical record of these almost-forgotten institutions.

This book is a part of that effort.

No Offense Intended
A Directory of Historical Disability Terms

Natalie Kirisits
Douglas Platt
Thomas Stearns

Design by Rachel Gottorff
Publisher: Nancy Palumbo
Editor: James M. Boles

ISBN: 978-0-9845983-9-7
Library of Congress Control Number: 2013941644

Front cover: Baby Farming. A practice from the Victorian Era. Baby farms took in unwanted children for a fee. See page 50.

People Ink Press
in association with the
Museum of disABILITY History
3826 Main Street
Buffalo, New York 14226

Books in Abandoned History Series:

On the Edge of Town: Almshouses of Western New York
by Lynn S. Beman and Elizabeth Marotta

Dr. Skinner's Remarkable School for "Colored Deaf, Dumb, and Blind Children" 1857 – 1860
by James M. Boles, EdD, and Michael Boston, PhD

When There Were Poorhouses: Early Care in Rural New York 1808 – 1950
by James M. Boles, EdD

An Introduction to the British Invalid Carriage 1850 – 1978
by Stuart Cyphus

Abandoned Asylums of New England
A Photographic Journey by John Gray
Historical Insight by the Museum of disABILITY History

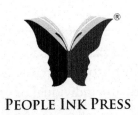

PEOPLE INK PRESS

Dedication

This book is dedicated to Georgiana Jungels for her inspirational leadership of the People Inc. Board of Directors and tireless service to those in need.

Table of Contents

Introduction

Terminology has always existed to describe and classify people with disabilities. The nature of these terms is dependent upon many factors—including the culture, beliefs, customs, and practices of an era. Consequently, they provide a means of examining how disabilities were perceived and treated during the period in which a term was used.

The *Directory of Historical Disability Terms* is the result of museum research into the history of early New York State almshouses, hospitals, institutions, and schools—along with notes of frequently asked questions from visitors to the Museum of disABILITY History in Buffalo, New York. Most of the terms were early practitioners' attempts to clarify and identify the nature and causes of diseases and deviations in human behavior. An attempt was made to include slang, including present-day terms, but the result was too toxic to print. As you read the directory, it is easily seen that, historically, yesterday's diagnosis can, a few generations later, become negative and enter everyday language.

Our main resources included the archives of the Museum of disABILITY History, the University at Buffalo's Health Sciences Library, and various digitized materials online. A note to readers: This directory is not intended to be a comprehensive dictionary of terms. It is a response to the need to provide students, museum visitors, and researchers with a glimpse into historic references that are connected to, and associated with, disabilities.

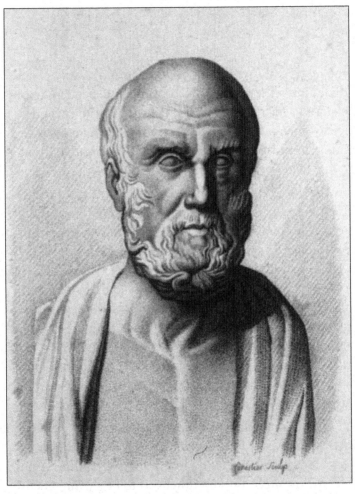

Hippocrates. Engraving by Ambroise Tardieu.

Chapter One:
Mental Health Terminology

Classification of mental health disorders appeared as early as the fifth century BCE, when Greek physician Hippocrates began to emphasize the importance of detailed observation in the treatment of patients. Hippocrates and his followers focused on discovering the natural causes of diseases instead of relying on theology or superstition. Environment, diet, and living habits were all considered during the process of diagnosis.[1] Hippocrates documented several types of mental disorders that we still recognize today—including mania, melancholia, and paranoia.[2]

The practice of Hippocratic medicine faded in the centuries following his death, and similar systems of classifying mental disorders did not appear until the Renaissance. Theology and superstition once again influenced people's perceptions of mental health. This changed after the late eighteenth century, as the formation of hospitals for the insane enabled physicians to conduct extensive observations on patients with "like symptoms" and thereby document patterns of mental disorders—along with the course of illnesses.[3] As psychiatry gradually matured into a scientific discipline, the "catalogues of nosology" (the classification of diseases) expanded accordingly.[4] Chapter One explores this period of clinical discoveries, along with obscure terms that related to mental health disorders.

Acromania – An incurable, violent form of mania with a high degree of motor activity.[5]

Aerumna – An old term applied to patients who displayed "weariness and unhappiness" (i.e., melancholia) due to suffering from a physical ailment.[6]

Agriothymia – Derived from the Greek, meaning "fierce disposition," the term denoted "furious insanity, maniacal furor"[7] and was used to describe patients who were considered dangerous and menacing; at one point synonymous with *homicidal insanity*. Physicians applied the diagnosis of *agriothymia ambitiosa*, also known as *Alexanderism*, to patients who displayed "an irrepressible desire to destroy or exterminate nations."[8] It received its name from Alexander the Great and his many military conquests.

Alcoholic Insanity – A term used to refer to the symptoms of mental derangement experienced by heavy consumers of alcohol following a "prolonged debauch."[9] Physicians noted changes in mood ranging from melancholia to acute mania, as well as the occurrence of illusions and hallucinations.[10] (cf. *Dipsomania*)

Alienist – A nineteenth-century term for physicians who specialized in the treatment of mental health disorders; that is, psychiatrists. They worked in hospitals for the insane. *Alienation* referred to the "separation" between oneself and the faculties of one's mind.

Amenomania – An obscure term created by American physician Benjamin Rush to denote a "form of partial insanity" characterized by an irrational sense of enthusiasm. Rush noticed the condition most frequently in "religious enthusiasts," some of whom believed that they were "the peculiar favorites of heaven, and exclusively possessed of just opinions of the divine will, as revealed in the Scriptures."[11]

Anomia – The "total absence" of a moral faculty; described in 1786 by Benjamin Rush, the founder of American psychiatry.[12] He later referred to it as "moral derangement."[13] According to Dr. Rush, a person's moral faculty could be affected by various factors— including climate, diet, drink, disease, idleness, excessive sleep, bodily pain, cleanliness, solitude, music, medicines, etc.

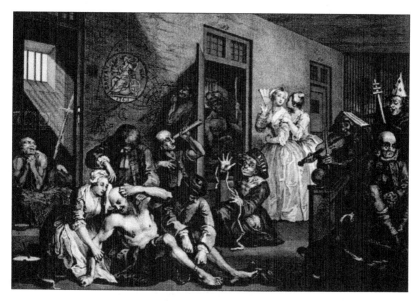

"The Interior of Bedlam" by William Hogarth. Date of Creation: 1735. This image depicts a cast of tormented characters inhabiting the famous Bethlem Royal Hospital. Two fashionable women appear in the background, having come to witness the antics of the insane as a form of entertainment.[14]

B

Bedlam – A euphemism for pandemonium or chaos, such as occurs in an insane asylum; derived from a "colloquial corruption" of the Bethlem Royal Hospital in London, England, which has functioned as a hospital for the mentally ill since 1547.[15]

Bell's Mania – An acute form of delirious mania described in 1849 by Dr. Luther V. Bell, superintendent of the Mclean Asylum for the Insane in Somerville, Massachusetts.[16] Patients experienced a sudden onset of the illness "without any precursory symptoms" and displayed "extreme violence," "intellectual wandering," and an "entire loss of appetite," along with hallucinations involving "impressions of sinfulness and personal danger."[17] About three-quarters of the cases that Dr. Bell examined died within two or three weeks—owing to extreme exhaustion—while the remainder "promptly and entirely recovered."[18] Because the combination of symptoms was so unlike anything else previously observed, Dr. Bell believed that it was an "overlooked and hitherto unrecorded malady."[19]

C

Chiromania – A common nineteenth-century term used to describe a relationship between masturbation and insanity. One author described in detail how a boy might adopt the habit at an early age and then continue the practice through adolescence and into adulthood until arriving at a moment where:

> *The idea of self-abuse haunts him wherever he goes and in whatever he is engaged. He loses his ability to resist the promptings of the baneful passion, and seeks every opportunity to reproduce the pleasurable sensations. The constant draughts made upon the*

nervous energies bring exhaustion and irritability upon the whole corporeal organization, and it is not long before the ensnared victim exhibits mournful evidence of declining health, as a matter of course.[20]

Cerebria – An early nineteenth-century term used by French psychiatrist Philippe Pinel to classify mental derangement in general.[21] He applied the diagnosis of *acute cerebria* to patients exhibiting mania, whereas *chronic cerebria* denoted patients exhibiting idiocy (which was considered a permanent, unimprovable condition at the time).

Compulsive Insanity – A psychopathic condition in which a patient experienced a "morbid persistence" of ideas or fears that interfered with their thoughts and actions.[22] Any compulsive acts that resulted were "accompanied by consciousness of the nature of the act, by feelings of anxiety, and by attempts at resistance."[23] (cf. *impulsive insanity*)

Cyclothymia – Derived from the Greek words *kyklos*, meaning "circle," and *thymos*, meaning "anger," German psychiatrist Karl Ludwig Kahlbaum introduced the term in 1882 to describe a condition signified by alternating moods of depression and joyfulness and "notable for its frequent periods of normality."[24] (cf. *manic-depressive insanity*)

Démence Précoce – A term coined by French alienist Benedict-Augustin Morel in 1853 to describe a psychotic disorder that affected primarily males in their young adulthood; characterized by a progressive degeneration of emotional and cognitive processes.[25] German psychiatrist Emil Kraepelin popularized the

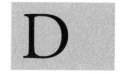

Latin translation *Dementia Praecox* at the end of the nineteenth century; however, his conception of the term differed from that of Morel, for he viewed it as "a series of states, the common characteristic of which is a peculiar destruction of the internal connections of the psychic personality." "Emotional and volitional spheres of mental life" were most prominently affected.[26] German psychiatrist Eugen Bleuler reclassified the condition as *schizophrenia* in 1911.

Dementia Infantilis – A term first used by Austrian educator Theodore Heller in 1908 to describe children who experienced sudden mental deterioration in early childhood—accompanied by a loss of speech and the regression of various cognitive abilities; currently known as *Childhood Disintegrative Disorder* or *Heller's Syndrome*.[27]

Demonomania – A belief that one is in communication with spiritual entities, accompanied by the sensation of being "controlled by and possessed by demons."[28] French psychiatrist Jean- Étienne Dominique Esquirol described several cases of demonomania in his 1838 *Treatise on Insanity*. One of which, a fifty-seven-year-old mother of fifteen, was admitted to the Salpêtrière Hospital in Paris shortly after throwing herself from a window. Esquirol made these observations upon her admission: "Expression of countenance restless. [Her] whole body is in a sort of vacillation and continual balancing. She is constantly walking about, seeking to do mischief."[29] She avoided her companions for fear that she would do them harm, "[talked] to herself, [saw] the devil on every side, and often [disputed] with him." He recorded her as saying:

For a million years I have been the wife of the devil . . . I have committed every kind of crime; have slain and robbed. The devil is continually telling me to slay, and even to strangle my children. In one minute, I commit more crimes than all rouges have committed in one hundred years . . . Hence I am not sorry to wear a strait waistcoat; for without this precaution, I should be dangerous.[30]

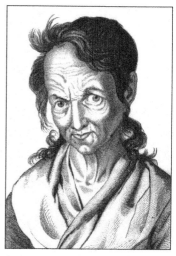

A woman who displayed symptoms of demonomania; engraving by Ambroise Tardieu. WELLCOME LIBRARY, LONDON.

Dereistic Thinking – Swiss psychiatrist Eugen Bleuler introduced this term in 1912 to describe "a form of fantasy thinking" common in patients with schizophrenia.[31] Bleuler derived the word *dereistic* from two Latin words meaning "away from reality,"[32] observing that these patients "often [lived] in an imaginary world of . . . wish fulfillments and persecutory ideas."[33] Dereistic Thinking follows "illogical, idiosyncratic reasoning"[34]—resembling what occurs in dream states.[35] Dr. Bleuler also termed it "autistic thinking."[36]

Dipsomania – Derived from the Greek words *dipsa*, "thirst" and *mania*, "madness," this nineteenth-century term denoted a morbid, irresistible desire for alcoholic drinks. One contemporary physician described the standard course of the condition as follows:

There is nausea, languor, vertigo . . . trembling of the limbs, [and] general malaise. After some days

. . . the appetite vanishes, sleep is disturbed, life appears intolerable. The image of the drink . . . presents itself then to the mind of the unfortunate; it so occupies his mind that he can receive no other impression, nor take heed to the advice of friends, or of their tears. The unfortunate feels himself forced of necessity to drink, and he says that if they do not furnish him drink he will become insane. Under the influence of this terrible impulse he places the lips to the cup and intoxicates himself at the first draught.[37]

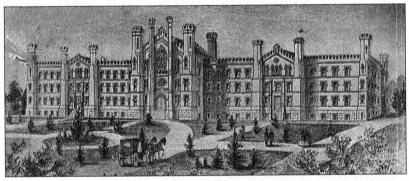

New York State Inebriate Asylum: a Gothic Revival limestone building inspired by European cathedrals and American insane asylums. Lavishly appointed inside and out, "its castellated façade, topped with turrets, towers, and buttresses, was spread across five attached buildings for nearly 1,500 feet." (John Crowley, "The Castle of Cures," *New York State Archives*, vol. 4, no. 4 (Spring 2005), 12–15).

In response to the appeals of Joseph Edward Turner, a physician-reformer who insisted that inebriety represented a clinical disease rather than a sin or "moral failing," New York established the world's first inebriate asylum in 1864. Located in Binghamton, the asylum provided care and medical treatment for what is now regarded as alcoholism—in a setting where "the self-destroying victim of intemperance could be restored to reason and usefulness, once more clothed in his right mind and [able] to bring light, joy, and peace . . . to the family circle."[38]

Furibundus – An old Latin word meaning "out of one's wits" with anger and fury.[39] Physicians applied the term to insane patients who were "maniacal, mad, [and] raging."[40] The term also appeared in a common maxim of law: *semel furibundus, semper furibundus praesumitur* (Once shown to be insane, always presumed to be insane)—which recognized mental incapacity to stand trial for crimes committed while under the sway of insanity.

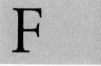

Hebephrenia – A classification introduced by German psychiatrist Ewald Hecker in 1871 "to represent [psychotic] conditions that began in adolescence, usually starting with a quick succession of erratic moods, followed by a rapid enfeeblement of all functions, and finally progressing to an unalterable psychic decline."[41] Patients displayed inappropriate, silly mannerisms and regressive behavior—with a tendency toward "smiling, laughter, and grimacing."[42]

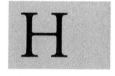

Hospitalism (or Anaclitic Depression in Its Sub-Lethal Form) – A pediatric diagnosis commonly used during the 1930s to describe infants who wasted away in the hospital. The term appeared as early as the late nineteenth century and was recognized by some as "a disease more deadly than pneumonia or diphtheria."[43] The term was also used by psychoanalyst René Spitz in 1946 to describe the condition of apathy and depression that appeared in infants who were deprived of emotional contact from their mothers. Spitz recorded some of his research on film and released

Psychogenic Disease in Infancy as an informational video in 1952—wherein he explained:

> [These infants] become lethargic, their motility retarded, their weight and growth arrested. Their face becomes vacuous; their activity is restricted to atypical, bizarre finger movements. They are unable to sit, stand, walk or talk.[44]

Hurry of the Spirits – An eighteenth-century term used to denote madness; quoted by English physician William Battie in his 1758 *Treatise on Madness*—one of the first books that focused on the treatment of mental health disorders.

I

Impulsive Insanity – A nineteenth-century term applied to any psychopathic condition in which "impulses [sprung] suddenly into consciousness and acts [followed] at once without the patient being able to resist them."[45]

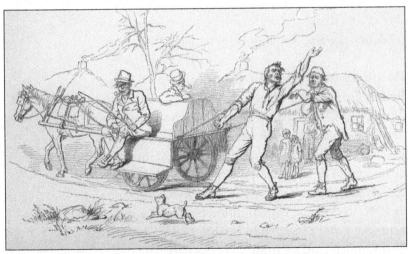

Taking Lunatics to Dublin in the Early Part of the Nineteenth Century.

Involution Melancholia – A type of melancholia that occurred after middle life—characterized by morbid depression, despondency, delusions of self-unworthiness, anxiety, agitation, and suicidal tendency.[46]

Lunatic – A generic term that was applied to people with mental health disorders, derived from the supposed influence of the moon in precipitating paroxysms of insanity (the Latin word *luna* referred to "the Goddess of the Moon" and *tic* meant "struck").[47] Though some physicians disagreed that lunar phases effected such profound changes, hospitals for the insane were known as lunatic asylums until the late nineteenth century.[48]

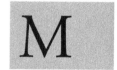

Mad-House – A popular nickname given to hospitals for the insane. This arose from the supposition that all people in such facilities were maniacs that could always be found "jabbering inanities, or shouting verbal nonsense, or muttering incoherent sentences."[49]

Manic-Depressive Insanity – A term introduced by German psychiatrist Emil Kraepelin to describe a group of mood disorders in which acute attacks of mania and depression "more or less" alternate with periods of relative normality, where few symptoms exist.[50] During the manic phase, Kraepelin's patients experienced "flight of ideas" (where ideas arose so fast that they found it difficult to express their thoughts and actions),[51] "exalted mood, and pressure of activity."[52] During

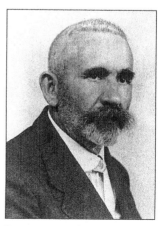

Emil Kraepelin.

the depressive phase, his patients experienced "sad or anxious moodiness and also sluggishness of thought and action," with some single idea long persisting in their mind.[53] These two "opposed phases" inspired the term. Kraepelin noted that some patients also experienced "states of the most profound confusion and perplexity," along with "well-developed delusions," leading him to infer that this group of mood disorders presented a "very varied character and composition."[54]

Menstrual Insanity – A nineteenth-century term applied to mental disturbances that appeared in some women before, during, or after the process of menstruation; "manifested clinically in the form of a psychosis like mania, less frequently melancholia, or as delirium."[55]

Monomania – A term introduced in the early nineteenth century by French psychiatrist Jean-Étienne Dominique Esquirol that denoted "a form of partial delirium"[56] characterized by preoccupation with a single fixed idea, or a single series of ideas, in an otherwise sound mind (from the Greek *monos*, "one," and *mania*, "madness").[57] Dr. Esquirol equated this delirium to an extremely passionate person who is unable to divert his or her thoughts from a particular idea.[58]

The officers of the New York State Lunatic Asylum at Utica described an instance of "epidemic monomania" that occurred in the mid-1840s when an American Baptist preacher named William Miller prophesied the second coming of Christ and the "immediate destruction of the world."[59] His apocalyptic vision spread through publications and a legion of proselytizers—some of whom became so delirious that they "forsook their respective callings, closed their shops and stores, [and] left their families to suffer" in order to attend meetings for "prayers and exhortations."[60]

With increasing numbers of adherents "swallowed up in the Maelstrom of Millerism," the rosters of lunatic asylums swelled with individuals who had lost their power of reason.[61] The officers at the Utica asylum observed that:

> *The greatest number of such cases occur among those who have long been pious, but who having become excited, agitated, and worn down by attendance, week after week, on nightly religious meetings, until their health became impaired; they then began to doubt their own salvation, and finally despaired of it, and becoming decidedly deranged, were conveyed by their beloved friends to our care, and often to prevent self-destruction.*[62]

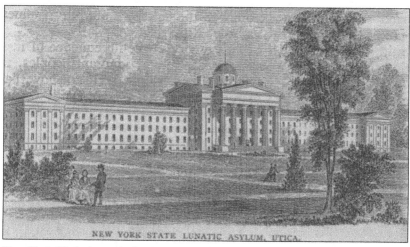

New York State Lunatic Asylum, Utica.

Moral Treatment – In the closing years of the eighteenth century, a few nonconformists commenced an intellectual revolution in the treatment of people with mental health disorders—known as "moral treatment." Removing mechanical restraints and forbidding violent punishments, the *doctrine of moral treatment* advocated a more compassionate approach to providing care—signified by intimate doctor-patient relationships and individualized recovery plans.[63]

These nonconformists derived inspiration from the Enlightenment ideals of social welfare and individual rights and instituted their reforms in various countries—almost entirely without knowledge of each others' efforts. Of particular note were Italian physician Vincenzo Chiarugi, French physician Philippe Pinel, English Quaker William Tuke (and his grandson Samuel Tuke), and American physician Benjamin Rush.

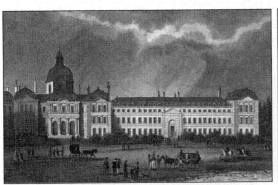
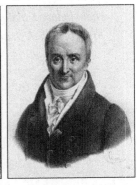

Salpêtrière Hospital for the Insane, located in Paris.　　　Philippe Pinel.

Pinel established a humane psychological approach to patient care that focused on therapy through proper diet and hygiene, physical and mental exercises (to keep the mind occupied), and the creation of a constant friendly atmosphere.[64]

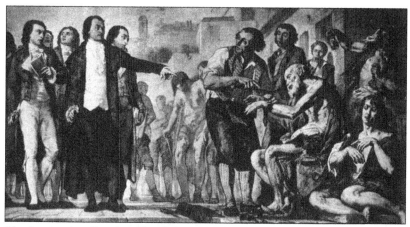

Pinel removing the shackles from patients at the Bicêtre Asylum.

According to an account written by his son, Pinel appealed to government officials at the height of the French Revolution—seeking to institute "moral treatment" at the Bicêtre Asylum in Paris. They responded, "Citizen, are not you yourself mad to think of unchaining such animals?" However, Pinel persisted and ultimately secured approval for his experiment. The first patient that he unchained was an old English captain who had been manacled for over forty years. He was considered the "most ferocious of all" for having once killed an attendant with a single blow; Pinel nevertheless entered the captain's cell and explained his desire to unchain the old man, under the condition that he would be "reasonable and . . . injure no one."[65] The captain agreed and, after several hours of attempting to stand up—for he had not used his legs in a long time—he finally regained enough strength and tottered toward the door. "His first movement was to look up at the heavens and to cry out in ecstasy, 'How beautiful!'" This feeling of rapture remained with him the entire day and at nightfall he returned "of his own accord to his cell [and] slept tranquilly."

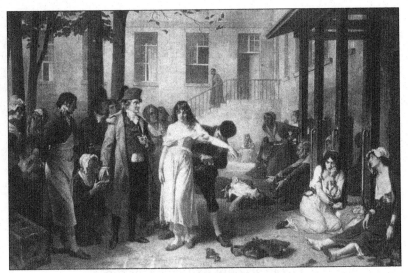

"Pinel at the Salpêtrière," painting by Robert Fleury.

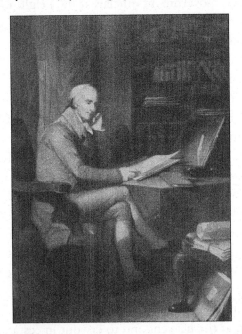

Dr. Benjamin Rush—often referred to as "The Father of American Psychiatry"— advocated for moral treatment and therapy in the United States during the mid eighteenth to early nineteenth centuries.

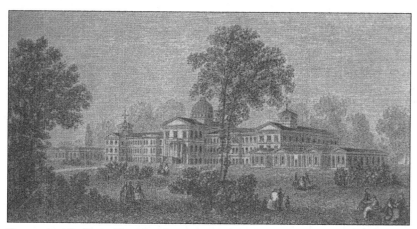

Pennsylvania State Hospital for the Insane, where Benjamin Rush served as primary physician. During his tenure, Rush brought the managers' attention to the lack of heating and ventilation in the cells and composed appeals to introduce opportunities for patient employment.[66]

During the nineteenth century, subsequent physicians and reformers developed the early ideas of moral treatment into a comprehensive ideology—the essentials of which were summarized by Amariah Brigham, superintendent of the New York State Lunatic Asylum at Utica from 1842–1849:

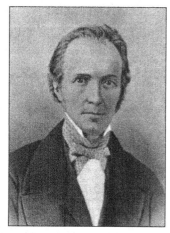

The removal of the [patient] from home and former associations, with respectful and kind treatment under all circumstances, and in most cases manual labor, attendance on religious worship on Sunday, the establishment of regular habits and of self-control, diversion of the mind from morbid trains of thought.[67]

Amariah Brigham (1798–1849).

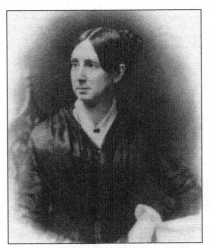

Dorothea Lynde Dix (1802–1887).

Dorothea L. Dix was a mid-nineteenth-century social reformer who visited almshouses, jails, and insane asylums across the United States in an effort to expose abysmal conditions. She presented her findings to members of state legislatures and insisted that systems of moral treatment be established at all facilities that provided care for the "mentally ill." Most of her knowledge on the subject came from her own personal investigations and through consulting with experts on moral treatment—including physicians Amariah Brigham, Luther V. Bell, and John S. Butler.[68]

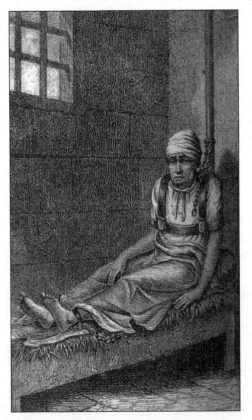

An etching of "Norris in Chains" depicted the outmoded, inhumane methods of caring for the insane—i.e., chains and bars for full restraint. The doctrine of moral treatment sought to abolish this type of "care."

Paresis (also known as *general paralysis of the insane* or *paralytic dementia*) – is a neuropsychiatric disorder that appears in the final stages of syphilis infection, affecting both the brain and central nervous system.

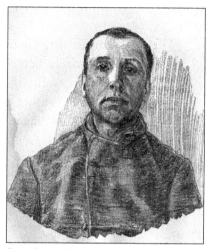

A patient with paresis.

French physician Antoine Bayle first identified paresis in 1822 as "a discrete disease entity characterized by speech impairment, weakening of motility in the arms and legs, and a delirium degenerating into dementia."[69] His discovery occurred after he performed autopsies on several patients who had displayed these symptoms and observed a "chronic inflammation of the meninges" (the system of membranes that envelops and protects the central nervous system).[70] This inflammation, Bayle argued, placed an increasing amount of pressure on the brain and caused the various symptoms to worsen as the disease progressed.[71] Physicians connected these symptoms to syphilis in the early nineteenth century.

Periodical Insanity – A term applied to the recurrence of insanity at regular intervals, separated by periods of "apparent mental soundness."[72]

Puerperal Insanity – A nineteenth-century term that denoted a link between insanity and the process of child-bearing. Many physicians believed that women could become insane at any point during the three "physiological phases" of pregnancy, childbirth, and lactation—reasoning that the "remarkable change in the functions of the nervous system" that occurred during these phases exposed women to extreme mental and physical exhaustion and left them susceptible to symptoms of derangement.[73]

T**ranquilizing Chair** – A method of restraining patients with mental health disorders developed by American psychiatrist Benjamin Rush in the late eighteenth century. The device aimed to restrict patients' movements and reduce their sensory stimulation[74] in a way that reflected more humane methods of care—such as those expounded by "moral treatment."

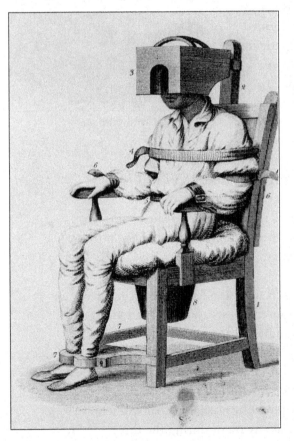

Tranquilizing Chair.

Chapter Two:
Intellectual, Cognitive, and
Developmental Disability Terms

Terminology related to intellectual, cognitive, and developmental disabilities evolved in a peculiar manner. During the mid-nineteenth century, physicians classified these various types of disabilities under a single clinical diagnosis known as "idiocy." People with significant intellectual impairments suffered from the "condition of idiocy" and prevailing opinion held that they were incapable of benefiting from education. Jean-Étienne Dominique Esquirol, head psychiatrist at the Salpêtrière Hospital in Paris, formulated this medical definition of idiocy in 1838:

> *Idiocy is not a disease, but a condition in which the intellectual faculties are never manifested or have never been developed sufficiently to enable the idiot to acquire such an amount of knowledge as persons of his own age, and placed in similar circumstances with himself are capable of receiving. Idiocy commences with life or at that age which precedes the development of the intellectual and affective faculties, which are from the first what they are doomed to be during the whole period of existence.*[75]

However, just a few years later, one of Esquirol's understudies—a teacher named Édouard Séguin—earned recognition for developing the first systematic approach to educating people with "idiocy," known as the "physiological method

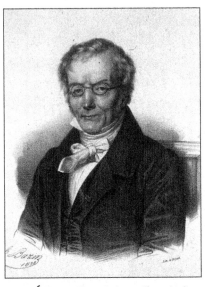

Jean-Étienne Dominique Esquirol.

of education." Séguin insisted that "idiocy" was not a fixed condition beyond means of improvement. Rather, he perceived "idiocy" as resulting from an "infirmity in the central nervous system, in which the organs and faculties of the child are separated from the normal control of the will, leaving [them] controlled by instincts and separated from the moral world."[76]

This, in turn, arrested normal development and caused the various deficiencies present within the person's mind and body. Séguin acknowledged that physical factors could complicate the educational process but maintained that people with "idiocy," similar to all other people, had "sensations, sentiments, and perceptions"—these were merely undeveloped.[77] To awaken these faculties, Séguin employed exercises that strengthened the muscular system and helped develop sensory perception and acuity. With time and effort, his students gained conscious control over their wills.

During the 1840s and 1850s, institutions for "idiots" started appearing in Europe and the United States—following the creation of the physiological method of education. In much the same way that hospitals for the insane enabled physicians to identify patterns of mental health disorders, these "idiot schools" enabled the classification of different sub-types of "idiocy"— especially due to the fact that physicians often occupied the role of superintendent.

This chapter examines some of the terms that were subsequently formulated—along with general terms related to intellectual, cognitive, and developmental disabilities.

A note to the reader: The entries provide historical snapshots and are not intended to be comprehensive definitions.

Amaurotic Family Idiocy – (now known as Tay-Sachs disease) this term first appeared in 1887 when Bernard Sachs, a neurologist at the Mount Sinai Hospital in New York, presented his research on a syndrome of infantile cerebro-macular degeneration,[78] which he believed to be genetically transmitted. The following description of the disease appeared in an early twentieth-century pediatric textbook:

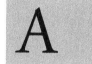

> *The onset . . . is usually observed in the second year. The child, hitherto healthy, cheerful, and well-developed, becomes quiet and sleepy while the attentive parent notices the beginning of an impairment of vision . . . . With the rapidly increasing loss of sight, to which deafness is usually added, a rapid deterioration of all the mental functions, approaching complete idiocy, makes its appearance. Simultaneously, a progressive muscular weakness develops . . . until they present the picture of complete bilateral paralysis . . . . The child dies by the end of the second or third year of life.*[79]

Ament – A person without a mind; an idiot.

Amentia – A Latin term meaning "absence of mind;" synonymous with mental deficiency. Scottish physician William Cullen composed one of the earliest definitions in 1777, viewing it as "imbecility of the judging faculty with inability to perceive or remember."[80] He classified three distinct types, based on whether the condition originated in birth, from a traumatic brain injury, or in old age.[81]

Anoia – A Greek term meaning "without mind," the term indicated a lack of understanding and was used to denote mental deficiency; especially idiocy.[82]

Backward Children – An early twentieth-century term applied to children who exhibited delayed development due to various causes (inherited or acquired) and "[could] never keep up with [their] fellows."[83] In a 1920s book on *mental abnormality*, the general characteristics of backward children were listed as: "dreaminess, stolidness, nervousness, excitability, and the inability to socialize."[84]

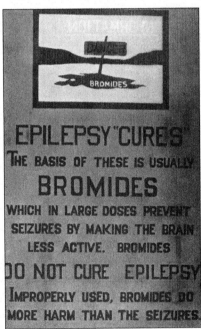

A "warning against the use of bromides," published in the *Twenty-Second Annual Report* of Craig Colony, 1916.

Borderland (or Borderline) – Physicians used this term to denote conditions which "[differed] from the normal but not sufficiently enough to involve a change in personality . . . or general and permanent mental inadequacy" (that is, feeble-mindedness).[85]

Bromism – In the late nineteenth- and early twentieth-century, a common form of treatment for people with epilepsy involved the administration of potassium bromide,[86] a type of salt with anticonvulsant and sedative properties that suppressed seizures and fits in the short-term but would cause "a great deal of harm" to a person's health when used for extended periods—a condition known as *bromism*.[87] Physicians at the Craig Colony for Epileptics in Sonyea, New York, observed that patients who displayed signs of *bromism* were "stupid, dull, and [seemed] bordering on dementia." They had no energy for work and were "perfectly listless."[88]

Changeling – An old term from Western European folklore, a changeling was a child substituted for another; an elf. An abnormal child was believed to be a changeling, especially if he or she had a physical or intellectual disability.

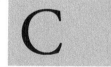

Cretinism – A medical term that originated in the eighteenth century to denote a condition of severely stunted physical and mental development resulting from thyroid deficiency.[89] The derivation is uncertain; however, most contemporary writers regarded it as "a corruption of the French *Chrétien*" (meaning Christian), "as indicative of the incapacity of these unfortunate beings to commit sin," as well as of the idea that they were still capable of accepting Christ's teaching and thus should be treated with kindness.[90] In

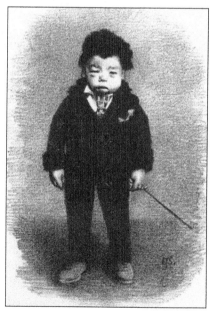

A cretin child.

1842, a physician named Johann Jakob Guggenbuhl established a treatment colony for cretins upon the slope of the Abendberg mountain in Switzerland, "about four thousand feet above [sea level]," and "to this elevated and healthful location he brought as many cretin children as he had the means of instructing."[91]

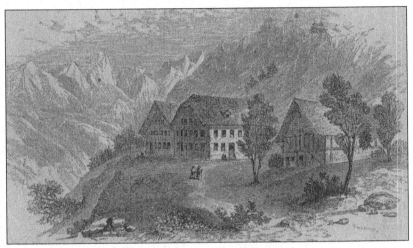

Treatment colony for cretins; Abendberg, Switzerland.

Defective Delinquent – A term introduced in the early twentieth century, applied to *mental defectives* who showed a propensity toward unsocial acts and criminal behavior.[92] New York established an institution for male defective delinquents at Napanoch in 1921 (and at Woodbourne in 1935) after prison and reformatory administrators began to report increasing numbers of feeble-minded in their institutions (evidenced by intelligence testing). A physician at Napanoch explained *defective delinquents* in the following manner:

. . . [They are] less able to appreciate the differences between right and wrong, and so [are] less likely to be deterred from wrongdoing by conscientious scruples . . .. [They are] less able to appreciate the dangers of detection and punishment to which [they expose themselves] when [they commit] a crime, and so [are] less likely to be deterred by fear . . . [and they are] apt to be suggestible and lacking self-control.[93]

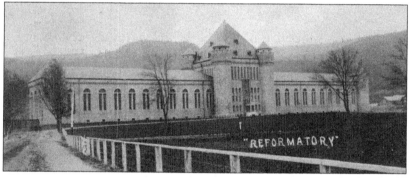

Institution for Defective Delinquents at Napanoch; regarded as the first institution of its kind in the country. The main building (pictured above) previously functioned as the "Eastern New York State Reformatory."

Facilities were also established for female defective delinquents; in 1920, a small section of the New York State Reformatory for Women at Bedford Hills began receiving patients. Later, in 1931, the Albion State Training School "was given over to the use of this group and renamed the Institution for Mentally Defective Women."[94]

Feeble-Minded – A generic term that appeared in the mid-nineteenth century to classify someone who was "unable to learn, think, work, [and] live in a normal way."[95] Application of the term was based on

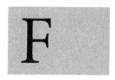

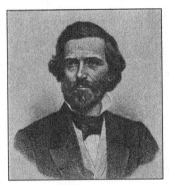
Samuel Gridley Howe.

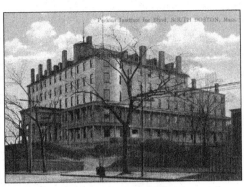
Perkins Institute for the Blind.

a subjective analysis of the individual in question and did not seek to address the cause of their deficiency or formulate a prognosis.[96] Samuel Gridley Howe established the first state school for the feeble-minded in 1848, located in a special wing of the Perkins Institute for the Blind in Boston, Massachusetts.

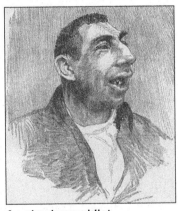
An almshouse idiot.

Fool – A term applied to any person lacking in judgment or prudence, or one who was deficient in common powers of understanding.

Charles Dickens summarized the subject by writing:
The main idea of an idiot would be of a hopeless, irreclaimable, unimprovable being.[97]

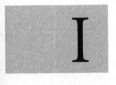

Idiocy – A term that encompassed all varieties of intellectual and cognitive disability. "Idiot" was derived from the Greek word *idios*, meaning "a peculiar or private person, one who is cut off from relationships with others and is alone"[98] (intellectual isolation).

Similar to the term *feeble-minded*, physicians applied the classification of *idiot* based on a subjective analysis of the person in question—it did not reference etiology or prognosis. Following the appearance of the Binet-Simon intelligence test in 1911, the term *idiot* became reserved for people who displayed the lowest grade of mental deficiency.

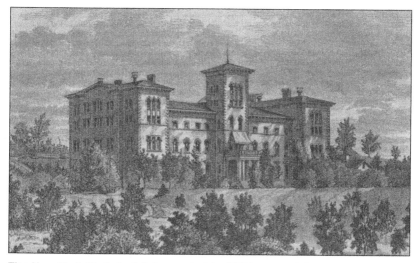

The New York State legislature voted in 1851 to establish an experimental school for "idiots"—the second institution of its kind in the United States and one of the first worldwide. Though the measure passed amid skepticism, favorable results led to the school securing permanent status in 1854. Located in Geddes, Syracuse, the New York State Asylum for Idiots (pictured above) inspired numerous other state legislatures to establish similar institutions. Dr. Hervey Backus Wilbur, a physician from Massachusetts, served as asylum superintendent from 1851 until his death in 1883.

Idiot Savant (now known as *Autistic Savant*) – A term applied to people who displayed prodigious abilities in one or more directions—which were exercised almost automatically and "[did] not seem to match their overall mental caliber."[99] *Savant* is French for *learned*.

The term *idiot savant* was introduced by British physician John Langdon Down in 1887.

He applied it to "[individuals] who, while feeble-minded, [exhibited] special faculties which [were] capable of being cultivated to a very great extent."[100]

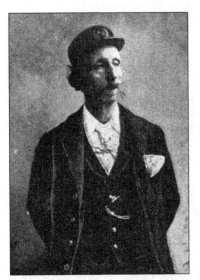

James Henry Pullen, an autistic savant patient at the Earlswood Asylum during Down's tenure, was affectionately known as "the Master Craftsman" for his "instinctive genius" in boat-building, engineering, and ivory-carving. Staff members at Earlswood, impressed by Pullen's talents, provided him with a special workshop filled with raw materials for his work.[101]

James Henry Pullen (1835 – 1916).

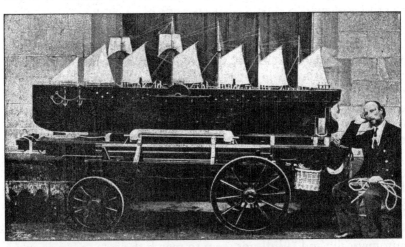

James Pullen exhibiting a replica of the Great Eastern.

Thomas "Blind Tom" Wiggins (1849–1908) was an African-American autistic savant and musical prodigy on the piano. Wiggins demonstrated enormous talent beginning in early childhood and became known for "his alleged ability to perform difficult selections almost flawlessly after one hearing, sing and recite poetry and prose in several languages, duplicate phonetically lengthy orations by noted statesmen, and reproduce sounds of nature, machines, and musical instruments on the piano."[102]

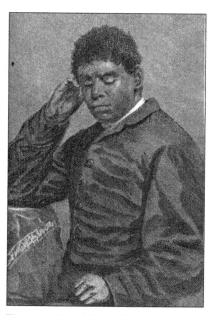

Thomas "Blind Tom" Wiggins.

Imbecile – A term that encompassed all varieties of intellectual and cognitive disability; derived "from the Latin *imbecillis*, 'weak' and *bacillum*, as 'needing a staff'; or *in vacillo*, 'tottering,' 'wanting strength of mind,' 'weak and feeble'; expressive of a certain degree of intelligence, but unstable, incapable, irresponsible."[103]

Innocents – An antiquated term applied to any person considered incapable of sin due to an absence of intellectual functioning. Such individuals were regarded as "eternal children" and therefore not responsible for their own actions.

Mental Defective – A generic term that appeared during the early twentieth century to classify individuals of subnormal intelligence who required

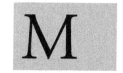

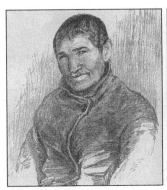

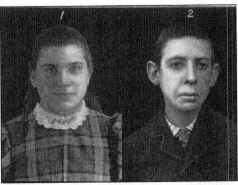

An imbecile.

1. Medium Grade Imbecile
2. High Grade Imbecile

special care and education in a state-sponsored institution (for the protection of themselves and of the community). The State of New York recognized *mental defectiveness* as "a condition of mind which is a departure from the general normal, but which is not a diseased condition or insanity."[104] The defining feature of mental defect was an inability to manage oneself or one's affairs. After 1919, state law permitted the incarceration of mental defectives, provided the person in question had an official "certificate of mental defect" completed by qualified examiners. However, because the law did not provide an objective measurement (a specific IQ point, for example), determination of mental defect was "subjective with the examiner."

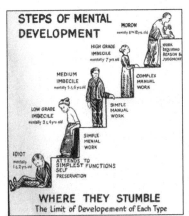

Early twentieth-century chart that depicts the "steps of mental development."

Mentally Deficient – A generic term that appeared in the late-nineteenth century; used to denote individuals who displayed below average intelligence—with an IQ between 70–75, and limited daily living skills (such as: the inability to communicate, care for oneself, or work).

Mongolian Idiocy – A term created by British physician John Langdon Down in 1866 after he observed that several of his patients at the Earlswood Asylum in England displayed strikingly similar clinical features to the extent that "when placed side by side," he found it "difficult to believe that they [were] not children of the same parents." Down's description of them appeared as follows:

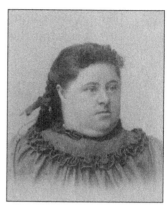

A woman with Down syndrome.

The face is flat and broad and destitute of prominence. Cheeks are roundish and extended laterally. The eyes are obliquely placed and the internal canthi . . . distant from one another. The lips are large and thick with transverse fissures. The tongue is long, thick, and much roughed. The nose is small.[105]

The term *Mongolian idiocy* was replaced by *Down syndrome* in 1961 after a group of genetic experts wrote the *Lancet* suggesting a more scientific, and less offensive, alternative.[106]

Moral Imbecile – Denoted a person who was morally blind, without morals; (synonymous with *defective delinquents*). Dr. Isaac Newton Kerlin, superintendent of the Pennsylvania Training School for Feeble-Minded Children from 1863 to 1893, observed that the "symptoms [of moral imbecility] . . . [were] confined either mainly or entirely to aberration of the 'moral sense,' with either no deterioration of the intellect or, if slight, such as could be considered secondary only." In fact, Kerlin remarked that many *moral imbeciles* exhibited precocious intelligence. He listed some of the behaviors that evidenced moral imbecility as follows:

> *Unaccountable and unreasonable frenzies . . .*
> *motiveless and persistent lying; thieving . . .*
> *a blind and headlong impulse toward arson;*
> *delight in cruelty . . . habitual willfulness and*
> *defiance, even in the face of certain punishment*
> *. . . and [mental dullness] or insensibility under*
> *disciplinary inflictions.*

In conclusion, Dr. Kerlin stated that "[their] aberrations are such as to make them the predestined inmates of our insane hospitals and jails." To reduce the chance of crime, Kerlin suggested methods of

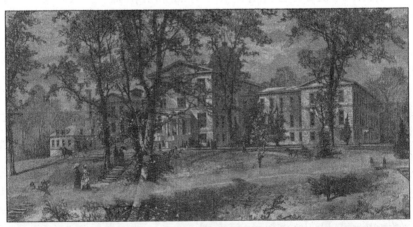

Pennsylvania Training School for Feeble-Minded Children. Superintendent Isaac N. Kerlin and his successor, Martin W. Barr, wrote extensively on the subject of "moral imbeciles."

training designed for their specific traits, "or, these failing, by their early and entire withdrawal from the community!"[107]

Morament – A term applied to low-grade morons who lacked the sense of morality. Physicians believed that "the moral center in the frontal lobe [was] organically disabled."[108]

Moron – Derived from the Greek word *moros*, meaning "dull," "stupid," or "foolish," American eugenicist Henry H. Goddard coined this term in 1910 to denote a new category of mental deficiency. It applied to a person with a mental age of eight or more, with an IQ of between 51 and 70, and was regarded as the highest grade of feeble-mindedness.[109] Morons were considered "intellectually dull, socially inadequate, and morally deficient."[110]

Natural – An idiot from birth; "[a person] on whom education can make no impression. As nature made him, so he remains."[111]

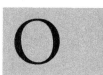

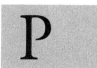

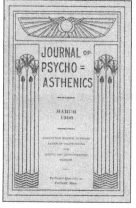

Journal of Psycho-Asthenics; March 1906.

Oligophrenia – A generic term that appeared during the late nineteenth century, signifying "weak-mindedness or mental deficiency."[112]

Psycho-asthenia – A term that appeared in the late nineteenth century to denote "feeble-mindedness" and "mental retardation." American physicians, educators, and researchers devoted to "the care, training, and treatment of the feeble-minded and of the epileptic" contributed numerous articles to the *Journal of Psycho-Asthenics,* which was published between the 1890s and the 1930s. These articles often contained the latest theories in the field and ideas for practical applications.

R

Railway Brain – A twentieth-century term that appeared in medical and legal reports to describe nervous disorders that resulted from railway accident-induced trauma. Claims against industrial companies became so numerous that people often "[questioned] the authenticity of the charges."[113] Some companies even hired law firms to investigate dubious cases. For example, New York neurologist Allan McLane Hamilton, "at the bidding of law firms, . . . shot motion picture films of . . . [alleged] trauma victims and analyzed their movements in hopes of discerning the subtle physiological differences between cases of faked and real traumas."[114]

S

Simpleton – A generic nineteenth-century term for a person lacking in common sense. Samuel Gridley Howe, superintendent of the Massachusetts Training School for Idiotic and Feeble-Minded Youth from 1848 to 1876, applied the term "simpleton" to denote people who showed a higher level of functioning than *idiots,*

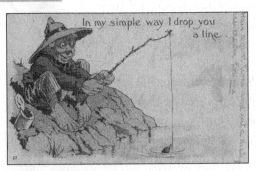

"Simple Jack."

imbeciles, or the *feeble-minded*, defining them as:

> . . . *the highest class of idiots in whom the harmony between the nervous and muscular system is nearly perfect; who consequently have normal powers of locomotion and animal action; considerable activity of the perceptive and affective faculties; and reason for their simple individual guidance, but not enough for their social relations.*[115]

Soft – A nineteenth-century term used to describe one who displayed low intelligence. It originated from the belief that people with intellectual impairments had brains that showed symptoms of softening. When Samuel Gridley Howe and other social reformers conducted an investigation into the condition of "idiots" within the State of Massachusetts (between 1845 and 1848), they observed that parents often administered peculiar methods in hopes of remedying their child's idiocy, one of which occurred as follows:

> *Sometimes [parents] find that the children seem to comprehend what they hear, but soon forget it; hence they conclude that the brain is too soft and cannot retain impressions, and then they cover the head with cold poultices of oak-bark, in order to tan, or harden, the fibers.*[116]

Un-Teachable Idiot – A term that appeared in the mid to late nineteenth century to denote "idiots" who were deemed incapable of benefiting from *any* methods of education—even those found at existing institutions for "idiots." In 1894, New York responded to a perceived increase of this class by

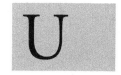

establishing the Custodial Asylum for Un-Teachable Idiots at Rome, New York. However, observation soon revealed that many patients at the asylum were capable of learning many useful skills and employing them with remarkable ability. Consequently, asylum superintendent Charles Bernstein sent the state legislature a request to remove the term "un-teachable idiot" from the institution's name and replace it with "custodial class of feeble-minded." In his first report as superintendent, Bernstein insisted:

> *The term 'un-teachable idiots' . . . [is] an unwarranted stigma on the lives of those poor unfortunates to so characterize them when as a matter of fact not one percent, if any, of our inmates are truly un-teachable.[117]*

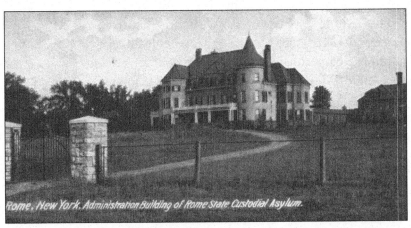

Rome, New York. Administration Building of Rome State Custodial Asylum.

Admin building, Rome State Custodial Asylum for Un-Teachable Idiots.

Chapter Three:
Physical Disability Terms

Blindman's Lantern – An old expression for "a walking stick with which a blind man guides his way; also known as '*Eyes to the Blind.*'"[118]

Camptocormia (also known as "bent spine syndrome") – an abnormal forward bending of the torso, "which increases during walking and abates in the recumbent position."[119] Derived from Greek words *kamptos* (meaning "bent") and *kormos* (meaning "trunk"),[120] French neurologist Alexandre-Achille Souques introduced the term during World War I to describe the bending posture of some soldiers returning from active service.[121] Because physicians discovered "no organic lesion" to account for the symptoms, it was regarded as "a hysterical phenomenon or conversion disorder"[122]—that is, a disorder presenting symptoms that cannot be explained by a comprehensive medical evaluation (often commencing suddenly after a stressful experience).

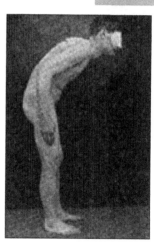

A soldier with camptocormia: Rosanoff-Saloff, "General Considerations on Camptocormia," Nouvelle iconographie de la Salpêtrière, vol. 28, no. 1 (1916–1917).

Charcot's Triad – A term applied to the most common clinical signs of multiple sclerosis, as observed by French neurologist Jean-Martin Charcot during his pioneering research at the Salpêtrière Hospital in the mid to late nineteenth century.[123] They include *dysarthria* (scanning speech), *nystagmus* (involuntary, rapid, and repetitive movement of the eyes), and *intention tremors* (involuntary trembling of the body).[124]

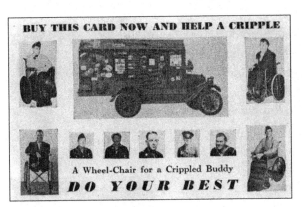

Charity card for "crippled" veterans; the front states, "Buy This Card Now and Help a Cripple."

Cripple – Now considered pejorative, this term appeared on the roster lists of almshouses and hospitals as recently as the mid-twentieth century to describe and classify people with physical or mobility impairments. The term even presented itself on charity cards whose proceeds were designed to benefit wounded United States veterans.

Freak – A pejorative term applied to any person of a strange demeanor or appearance. During the mid-nineteenth century, "freak shows" attained a large amount of popularity in the United States and Europe. They typically featured showmen and entertainers traveling to circuses, carnivals, and amusement parks in order to display human oddities for money. Coney Island in New York City often featured permanent

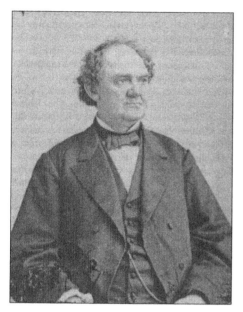

Phineas Taylor Barnum. American showman, scam artist, and entertainer, Barnum promoted an assortment of "freak shows" and established the circus that ultimately became the Ringling Bros. and Barnum & Bailey Circus.

displays of "freaks"—attracting tens of thousands of visitors annually.[125] Several broad categories of "freaks" existed:

- **Born freak** – a person with a natural physical anomaly, such as conjoined twins.
- **Gaffed freak** – a person who pretended to have a physical anomaly; also known as "fakes" or "phonies."
- **Made freak** – a person who modified their appearance in hopes of becoming unusual enough for an exhibit. For example, some acquired strange tattoos or grew their beards or hair exceptionally long.
- **Novelty act** – a person "who [did] not rely on any physical characteristics, but [could] perform an unusual act such as sword swallowing."[126]

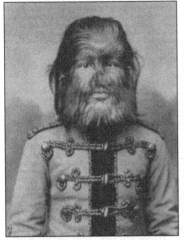

JoJo "the Dog-Faced Boy." Born with a rare condition known as hypertrichosis, the Russian boy attracted the attention of a circus and was brought to London, England, in 1884. Several years later, famous showman P.T. Barnum transported the boy to the United States, where he became one of the biggest "freak show" attractions. JoJo, whose real name was Fedor Jeftichew, displayed a significant amount of intelligence and spoke several languages. Hypertrichosis (also called "Ambras syndrome") is a rare condition that results in a considerable amount of hair growth on the body. Substantial cases have been called "werewolf syndrome," because the appearance is similar to the mythological werewolf.

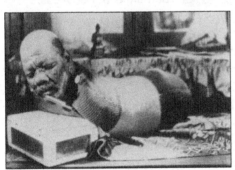

"Prince Randian." Reportedly from the West Indies, he was born without any arms or legs and became a star attraction at Coney Island for many years. Showmen introduced Prince Randian as the "human caterpillar who crawls on his belly like a reptile!" His trademark stunt involved rolling and lighting a cigarette using solely his lips. He starred in the 1932 movie *Freaks*.

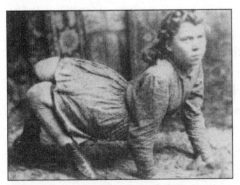

Pictured on the left is Lucy Elvira Jones. Double-jointed at the knees and elbows, she walked on all fours at "freak shows." Here, at the Dallas, Texas, State Fair in 1894, Lucy is only thirteen years old.

Giant – A term that has derivations from the old French word *geant*, as well as the Greek and Latin word *gigas*. The tall stature is due to excessive growth of the lower extremities, yet the head size and trunk are nearly the same size as a regular person of the same age.

Homunculus – A term that denotes a type of "little man; a dwarf without deformity of the spinal column or disproportion of extremities to trunk."[127]

Infantile Paralysis – An old synonym for *poliomyelitis*: an acute, infectious viral disease that can cause muscle weakness, physical paralysis, and even death. Thousands of people were paralyzed during "polio epidemics" in the late nineteenth and early twentieth centuries. American physicians Jonas Salk and Albert Sabin developed vaccines in the 1950s and '60s, facilitating the eradication of polio from most countries.

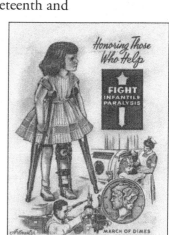

Various efforts initiated to combat infantile paralysis:

1. A child with partial paralysis due to poliomyelitis stands with crutches and a leg brace.

2. A nurse cares for a patient with poliomyelitis who requires an "iron lung" in order to breathe.

3. A scientist examines specimens through a microscope.

4. A dime, signifying the *March of Dimes* charity campaign — a U.S. nonprofit organization founded in 1938 by then-president Franklin Delano Roosevelt.

M

Microcephaly – A rare neurological disorder characterized by an abnormally small head—usually more than two standard deviations smaller than average for one's age and sex (with accompanying intellectual impairments). During the nineteenth and early twentieth centuries, some physicians believed that microcephaly represented "an instance of atavism"—that is, the reappearance of traits from some very remote ancestral type.[128] People with microcephaly were often called *pinheads*, as evidenced in P.T. Barnum's famous "Freak Shows."

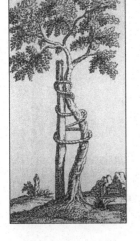

Microcephalics.

O

Orthopaedia – Derived from the Greek words *orthos* (meaning "straight" or "correct"), and *paideion* (meaning "child"), this term appeared in 1741 when French physician Nicolas Andry published *Orthopaedia: Or the Art of Correcting and Preventing Deformities in Children*. Andry advocated regular exercise to preserve the body's overall health and presented various methods of correcting spinal and bony deformities—such as the following procedure that aimed to reduce excessive inward curvature of a child's leg:

Apply, as soon as possible, a small plate of iron upon the hollow side of the leg and

Frontispiece of *Orthopaedia*, depicting the straightening of a tree.

fasten it about the leg with a linen roller. This roller must be made tighter and tighter every day 'till it compresses sufficiently the part that branches out . . . In a word, the same method must be used in this case, for recovering the shape of the leg, as is used for making straight a crooked trunk of a young tree.[129]

Paralysis Agitans – (now known as *Parkinson's disease*), is a degenerative disorder of the central nervous system that typically commences during middle or later life.[130] Symptoms include tremors (shaking), rigidity, slowness of movement (bradykinesia), stooping posture, shuffling gait (due to difficulty walking), and various speech disorders. English physician James Parkinson described the disorder in 1817 when he published *An Essay on the Shaking Palsy*. In the essay, Dr. Parkinson illustrated six patient cases—three of whom he personally examined; the rest he "noticed casually in the street."[131] None were able to suggest any circumstance that could account for their condition—most regarding it "as a mere consequence of constitutional debility;" i.e., a natural result of growing old.[132] Parkinson explained:

So slight and nearly imperceptible are the first inroads of this malady, and so extremely slow is its progress that . . . the patient can [rarely] form any recollection of the precise period of its commencement. The first symptoms perceived are, a slight sense of weakness, with a proneness to trembling in some particular part; sometimes in the head, but most commonly in one of the hands and arms . . . the propensity to lean forward becomes invincible. As the debility increases and the influence of the will over the muscles fades away, the tremulous agitation becomes more vehement.[133,134]

The disorder received more attention during the early 1860s when Jean-Martin Charcot performed further research and provided new descriptions of the symptoms.

Phthisis – A nineteenth-century term applied to tuberculosis of the lungs.[135]

Timber-Toe – An old term used to refer to a person with a wooden leg.[136]

T

Miscellaneous Terminology

Abram Men – A term applied to paupers who feigned insanity in order to beg alms.

Alice-in-Wonderland Syndrome – Described by British physician John Todd in 1955, this neurological condition leads people to experience alterations in their perception of time, space, and body image, as well as feelings of "de-realization, depersonalization, and somato-psychic duality" (or a separation of one's mind from one's body).[137] Symptoms appear in the course of a wide variety of disorders, "such as migraine, epilepsy, cerebral lesion, intoxication with [psychoactive] drugs, the deliria of fevers, [drowsy] states, and schizophrenia."[138] The term is a reference to the similar experiences of the character "Alice" in Charles L. Dodgson's 1865 book *Alice's Adventures in Wonderland*.

Illustration from *Alice's Adventures in Wonderland* by John Tenniel.

Almshouse – A synonym for poorhouse; a facility operated by the local government or a charity to house people in need of care—including those with physical, intellectual, and mental disabilities.

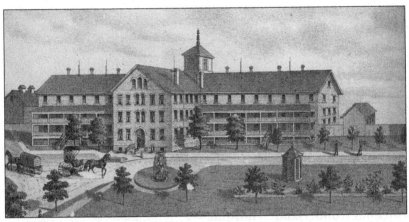

Erie County, New York Almshouse.

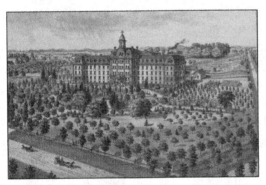

The Providence Lunatic Asylum was established in 1860 by physicians Austin Flint and James Platt White, with the help of the Sisters of Charity. The asylum opened in July 1861 at the corner of Main and Humboldt Park, Buffalo, NY. Sisters of Charity Hospital of Buffalo now occupies the site.

Asthenia – A term that denotes general debility; "loss of muscular energy and strength,"[139] often observed after disease or trauma.

Asylum – A safe place or haven, "isolated from the frenzy and disorder of the cities,"[140] that aimed to cure mental health disorders by bringing a quiet "discipline to the victims of a disorganized society."[141]

B

Baby Farming – A peculiar practice from the Victorian era that consisted of people taking in unwanted babies for a fee. These babies were often unwanted on account of illegitimacy or because they displayed a disability.

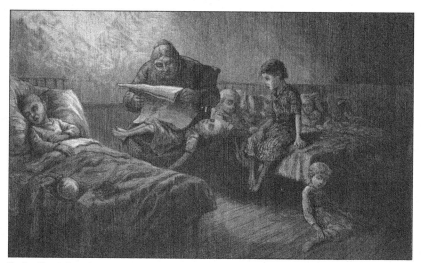

Baby Farming in New York; scene at an "asylum and sanitarium for children."

Some baby farmers abused the practice, adopting numerous children who were then neglected to the point of serious deficiencies and in some cases death.

Catalepsy – A condition that occurs in a variety of physical and psychological disorders, characterized by lack of response to external stimuli and by muscular rigidity.

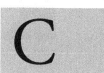

Dacrygelosis – A condition characterized by alternating spells of laughing and crying, seen most frequently in patients with schizophrenia.

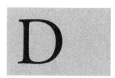

Destitute – Without means of subsistence; lacking food, clothing, and shelter; completely impoverished.

Disappointment Room – Families with financial means sometimes constructed a special room in their home to hide a disabled child. The room was locked on the outside and could include a center drain for human waste.

Dotard – A person weak-minded from old age or, more rarely, from disease or excess.[142] The term also appeared as *dotterel* and was contained in the phrase *to dor the dotterel*, which meant "to cheat the simpleton" (*dor* is an archaic word meaning to trick or cheat).[143]

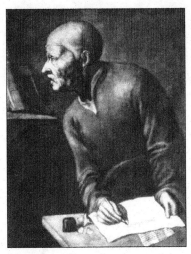

Dunce – A person of weak-intellect. The term is derived from a late-thirteenth-century philosopher-theologian named John Duns Scotus, known as "Doctor Subtilis" because of his penetrating and subtle manner of thought. However, later philosophers accused him of sophistry (presenting arguments that appear well-reasoned on the surface but are actually false). This led to the name *Duns* to become synonymous for "somebody who is incapable of scholarship."[144]

John Duns Scotus.

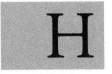

Happy Puppet Syndrome – (a pejorative term for *Angelman syndrome*) – In 1965, a British pediatrician named Harry Angelman described a rare neurogenetic disorder affecting several children who had been admitted to the Warrington General Hospital. They each displayed "severe intellectual disability, ataxia [loss of muscle coordination], absent speech, jerky arm movements, and bouts of inappropriate laughter."[145] Angelman later described how he conceived of the "happy puppet" terminology:

[These three children] had a variety of disabilities and although, at first sight, they seemed to be suffering from different conditions, I felt that there was a common cause for their illness. The diagnosis was purely a clinical one because . . . I was unable to establish scientific proof that the three children all had the same handicap. In view of this I hesitated to write about them in the medical journals. However, when on holiday in Italy I happened to see an oil painting in the Castelvecchio Museum in Verona called "a Boy with a Puppet." The boy's laughing face and the fact that my patients exhibited jerky movements gave me the idea of writing an article about the three children with a title of Puppet Children.[146]

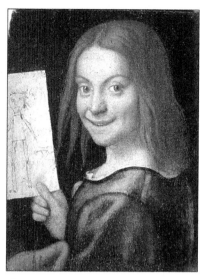

"Boy with a Puppet" by Giovanni Francesco Caroto.

Physicians engaged in genetic mapping during the 1980s discovered that the syndrome is caused by a partial deletion of the fifteenth maternal chromosome; it is often misdiagnosed as cerebral palsy or autism.

Infirmary – A place where the infirm or sick are lodged for care and treatment.

Marasmus – Extreme malnutrition and emaciation (especially in children); can result from inadequate intake of food, mal-absorption, or metabolic disorders.

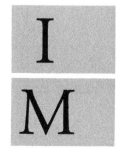

Mattoid – "A person of erratic [or abnormal] mind, a compound of genius and fool."[147] The term appeared in English in 1891 through a translation of the nineteenth-century Italian criminologist Cesaré Lombroso's work, *Man of Genius.*

Morotrophium – An old term for an asylum or hospital for the mentally ill.

O

Orthogenics – An antiquated term coined by American clinical psychologist Lightner Witmer to denote "the science of normal development." *Orthogenics* concerned itself primarily with "the causes and treatment of retardation and deviation" and examined "all the conditions which facilitate, conserve, or obstruct the normal development of mind and body."[148]

P

Periblepsis – An obscure term used to describe "the wild stare of a delirious person, with elements of bewilderment, consternation, and terror."[149]

Phrenology – A popular psychological theory of the 1800s, which held that measurements of the skull could be used to understand the interior of a patient's mind (that is, their mental characteristics).

Psychiatry – Derived from two Greek words meaning "healing of the mind," *psychiatry* refers to the body of knowledge pertaining to mental health disorders.[150]

Psychometric Test – "A laboratory test for determining the rapidity and accuracy of mental operations," such as the Binet-Simon intelligence test.[151]

Syndrome – "A group of clinical signs or symptoms which may result from diverse causes; therefore, it does not constitute a disease entity."[152]

Historical Snapshots of Modern Terminology (Mental Health Terms)

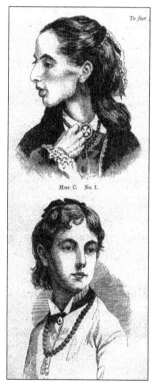

Image depicts "Miss C.," one of Dr. Gull's patients with anorexia nervosa, before and after her treatment. WELLCOME LIBRARY, LONDON.

Anorexia Nervosa –
English physician William W. Gull introduced this term in 1874 to describe a nervous disorder characterized by a patient's refusal to eat, thus resulting in extreme emaciation and a "depression of all the vital functions." He observed that the disorder occurred mostly in young women and believed that it resulted from "a morbid mental state" —similar to hysteria.[153]

Benign Stupors –
Introduced by Swiss psychiatrist August Hoch in the early 1900s to denote certain forms of manic-depressive psychoses that "mimicked the symptoms

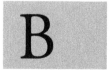

of the catatonic type of *Dementia Praecox*, but which did not have the poor prognosis."[154] Patients displayed "apathy, inactivity, mutism, catalepsy, and negativism;" Hoch wrote: "The law of benign stupor is a limitation of energy, emotion, and ideational content."[155]

C

Catatonia – A neuropsychiatric syndrome that appears in a diverse range of conditions. It is characterized by long periods of stupor, mutism, muscular tension, and negativism (a tendency to resist external and internal stimuli), and is occasionally punctuated by moments of extreme excitement.[156] German psychiatrist Karl Ludwig Kahlbaum introduced the term before an audience at the University of Konigsberg in 1868 and later published a monograph on the subject in 1874, titled *Catatonia or Tension Insanity*.[157]

D

Delirium Tremens – A term introduced by British physician Thomas Sutton in 1813 to describe the acute episode of delirium that occurs in people during their withdrawal from prolonged, heavy alcohol consumption.[158] Symptoms include body tremors, insomnia, agitation, confusion, visual and aural hallucinations, seizures, rapid heartbeat, profuse sweating, high blood pressure, and fever.[159] A description of these hallucinations appeared in one doctor's prize-winning dissertation on the subject, published in 1831:

> *[Delirium Tremens'] conspicuous attribute consists in a belief of the existence of frightful objects, in positions in which . . . it is . . . impossible for them to be situated . . . . The patient fancies that Satan is attached to the ceiling, and as his disease increases in*

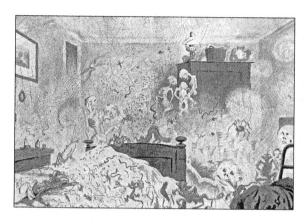

A patient's
representation of
the hallucinations
resulting from an
episode of Delirium
Tremens.

*intensity, his majesty appears to hover over him,
and he will shrink as if there were reality in the
impending danger .... The cooperation of his
attendants is frequently solicited to assist him
in defending himself against enemies . . . or to
drive from his presence disgusting objects that
annoy him exceedingly, such as snakes, lice, rats,
frogs, and vermin of every description, with
which he imagines the floor of his chamber or
his bed to be covered.*[160,161]

Dementia – A group of symptoms that indicate
a deterioration in mental functioning—including
memory loss, impaired judgment and language,
changes in personality, disturbances in thought,
anxiety, and difficulty with everyday activities and
experiences. Dementia can result from traumatic brain
injuries, strokes, infections, neurodegenerative diseases,
and old age.[162,163]

- **Alzheimer's Disease,** "a progressive and fatal
  disease of the brain,"[164] is the most common type of
  dementia, accounting for an estimated 60-80% of
  cases.[165] German psychiatrist and neuropathologist
  Alois Alzheimer identified the first case in 1906

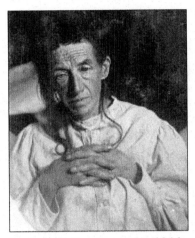

Auguste Deter, November 1902.

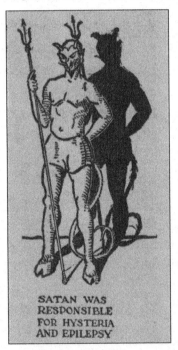

SATAN WAS
RESPONSIBLE
FOR HYSTERIA
AND EPILEPSY

after performing a brain autopsy on a former patient of his, a middle-aged woman named Auguste Deter who had come under his care in November 1901 at the Institution for the Mentally Ill and for Epileptics in Frankfurt, Germany. During the autopsy, he noticed plaques and neurofibrillary tangles in her brain—along with evidence of arteriosclerosis (degenerative changes in the arteries; characterized by thickening of the vessel walls and diminished blood circulation).

Her first "disease symptom" appeared in the form of "a strong feeling of jealously towards her husband . . . [and] very soon she showed rapidly increasing memory impairments; she was disoriented carrying objects to and fro in her flat and [often] hid them."[166] Part of Alzheimer's analysis involved asking Auguste simple questions and recording her responses. She displayed noticeable confusion and evidence of a relentlessly wandering mind— her speech being described

Historically, epilepsy was known as the *Sacred Disease* and people believed that seizures signified an attack from a demon. Even during the Age of Enlightenment, some physicians believed that epilepsy was caused by spiritual factors—attributing the symptoms to devils, demons, and witches.[167]

by Dr. Alzheimer as "spontaneous" and "full of paraphrasic derailments and perseverations" (the repetition of something in an insistent or redundant manner).

Epilepsy – A diverse set of neurological disorders characterized by seizures and "fits," accompanying loss of consciousness. The term is derived from the Greek word *epilēpsía*, meaning "to take hold of, to seize."[168] Prior to the late nineteenth century, many aspects of epilepsy remained an unsolved riddle to physicians, and few efforts were undertaken to provide relief for these people. Refuge could only be found in almshouses or, occasionally, hospitals for the insane —two environments "where the life, atmosphere, and diet were most unfitted for them."[169]

This changed following the discovery of a promising model of therapeutic care, which inspired

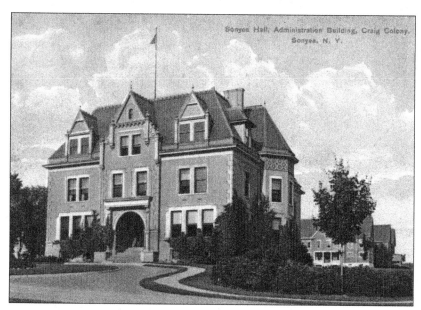

Administration Building, Craig Colony for Epileptics, New York.

New York State to establish the Craig Colony
for Epileptics in April 1894. This was the second
institution within the United States, and one of the
first worldwide, created for people with epilepsy—
and its success enabled a philanthropic movement to
"spread with marvelous and unprecedented rapidity
from the Atlantic to the Pacific."[170]

The physicians at Craig Colony aimed to
create a therapeutic environment where people with
epilepsy could receive access to care, education, and
labor opportunities. The colony's first superintendent,
Dr. William P. Spratling, closely adhered to the maxim
"*mens sana in corpora sano*," which translates, "a healthy
mind in a healthy body."[171] Ensuring that patients
received ample exercise, exposure to clean air, and an
appropriate diet as often as possible was considered
essential to improving their physical and mental
health.[172]

Hysteria – The term *hysteria* is derived from the Greek
word *hystera*, meaning "womb," and refers to a nervous
disorder characterized by heightened emotional states,
anxiety, and various mental alterations. Physicians long
believed that hysteria resulted from a "disturbance
in the womb,"[173] and thus confined the diagnosis
exclusively to women.[174] Because the symptoms could
accompany a variety of other nervous disorders,
hysteria was often applied to patients whose
condition was otherwise unexplainable.[175] Significant
advancements in the understanding of hysteria
occurred during the 1870s when a French neurologist
named Jean-Martin Charcot conducted an in-depth
study on three women admitted to the hysteria ward at
the Salpêtrière Hospital in Paris.[176]

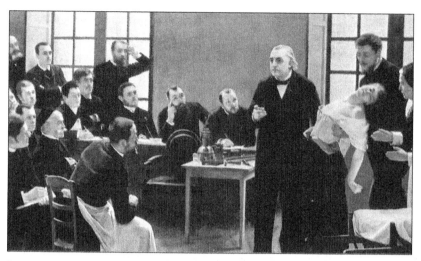

Dr. Jean-Martin Charcot shows his students a woman in a hysterical trance—while teaching at the Salpêtrière Hospital in Paris, France. Date of creation: 1887. Artist: André Brouillet.

Insane – A term that refers to someone who exhibits an unsoundness of mind; characterized by abnormal mental and behavioral patterns.[177] Dr. Amariah Brigham, the first superintendent of the New York State Lunatic Asylum at Utica, and editor of the *American Journal of Insanity*, defined it as: "A chronic disease of the brain, producing either derangement of the intellectual faculties, or prolonged change of the feelings, affections, and habits of an individual."[178]

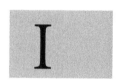

Mania – Derived from the Greek word for "madness" and "frenzy," nineteenth- and twentieth-century physicians used this term to denote abnormal levels of excitement during a period of pronounced psychosis. Esquirol, physician at the Salpêtrière Hospital in Paris, illustrated several characteristic changes that appeared in patients with acute forms of mania:

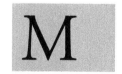

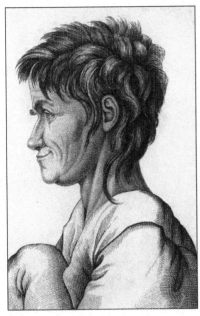

His actions are mischievous; and he desires to overthrow and destroy everything. He is at war with everybody; and hates all [which] he [formerly loved]. He is the very genius of evil, who delights in the confusion, disorder, and fear which he spreads around.[179]

Melancholia – In the nineteenth and early twentieth centuries, physicians used this term to denote a recurrent mood disorder that was characterized by a depressed, agonized state and dulled nervous functions. Cognition and perception were both affected. The patient experienced subdued emotions, wherein "everything [seemed] colorless and strange."[180] Association of ideas became languid and thinking "[revolved] monotonously [around] misfortune."[181] As one physician said of his melancholic patients:

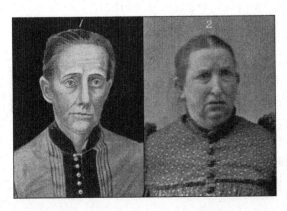

1: Simple Melancholia
2: Melancholia with agitation.

*There appears gradually a sort of mental sluggishness;
the patients find difficulty in coming to a decision and
in expressing themselves . . .. They fail to find the usual
interest in their surroundings . . .. They appear dull
and sluggish, and explain that they really feel tired and
exhausted.*[182]

Schizophrenia – Swiss psychiatrist Eugen Bleuler
introduced this term in 1911 to replace *dementia
praecox*, for he observed that the disorder "need not
always progress as far as dementia and [did] not always
appear *praecociter*," i.e., at a youthful age.[183]
He derived the term *schizophrenia* from the Greek
words "to split" and "mind"—explaining that the
disorder was characterized by a "split in psychic
functioning" (wherein a blurring of reality and fantasy
occurred), "alterations in the thinking process, and
disharmony of affect" (emotional imbalance).[184]
Ambivalence and autistic thinking (preoccupation with
one's inner thoughts) were also described as prominent
symptoms—along with varying degrees of delusions
and hallucinations.[185]

S

Historical Snapshots of Modern Terminology (Intellectual, Cognitive, and Developmental Disabilities)

Asperger syndrome – A developmental disorder situated within the autism spectrum. It bears the name of Austrian pediatrician Hans Asperger, who identified the syndrome in 1944 while treating four unusual boys at the University Pediatric Clinic in Vienna. These boys, aged six to eleven, each presented "an abnormal personality structure"—typified by "severe difficulties of social integration" that overshadowed everything else. They displayed a notable lack of empathy and engaged in repetitive patterns of behavior —often becoming intensely absorbed in some particular topic.[186] Asperger called them "little professors" because of their ability to discuss their favorite subjects in great detail (and their propensity to

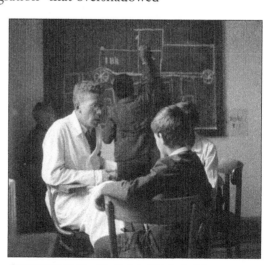

Asperger at the Pediatric Clinic in Vienna; circa 1940s.

speak "like an adult" at an early age). Fritz, one of the children examined by Asperger, arrived at the clinic after being declared "uneducable" at the end of his first day of school. Fritz failed to get along with any of the other classmates and, in fact, "was not interested in them"—for "they only 'wound him up.'" Furthermore, Fritz "did not know the meaning of respect and was utterly indifferent to the authority of adults."[187] Asperger observed that he "[gave] full rein to his internally generated impulses," noting:

> *His eye gaze was strikingly odd. It was generally directed into the void . . . . When somebody was talking to him, he did not enter into the sort of eye contact which would normally be fundamental to conversation. He darted short "peripheral" looks and glanced at both people and objects only fleetingly. It was "as if he wasn't there."*

Attention-Deficit Disorder – A behavioral disorder characterized by lack of attention, hyperactivity, and impulsive behavior. One of the earliest descriptions appeared in 1798 when Scottish physician Alexander Crichton identified a type of "mental restlessness:"

> *In this disease of attention . . . every impression seems to agitate the person, and gives him/ her an unnatural degree of mental restlessness. People walking up and down the room, a slight noise in the same, the moving of a table, the shutting of a door suddenly, a slight excess of heat or of cold, too much light, or too little light, all destroy constant attention in such patients, inasmuch as it is easily excited by every impression.[188]*

George Frederic Still, known as the Father of British Pediatrics, provided further insight in 1902 when he analyzed forty-three children who displayed an "abnormal incapacity for sustained attention." This rendered some of them "backward in school attainments," despite their appearing "as bright and intelligent as any child could be."[189]

Autism – A developmental disorder that appears in early childhood (prior to age three) and is signified by "impairments in socialization, communication, and imagination."[190] American psychiatrist Leo Kanner introduced the label *early infantile autism* in 1943 after observing a group of eleven children at the Johns Hopkins Hospital who displayed "a number of essential common characteristics"—the most conspicuous of which was "[their] inability to relate themselves in the ordinary way to people and situations from the beginning of life."[191] They engaged in restrictive and repetitive patterns of behavior and demonstrated "an insistence on sameness" in their surrounding environment. Everything that infringed upon this desire represented "a dreadful intrusion."[192]

Furthermore, they displayed "an all-powerful need for being left undisturbed"—a trait recognized early on by Kanner:

> *The children's relation to people is altogether different. Every one of [them], upon entering the office, immediately went after blocks, toys, or other objects, without paying the least attention to the persons present. It would be wrong to say that they were not aware of the presence of persons. But the people, so long as they left the child alone, figured in about the same manner*

*as did the desk, the bookshelf, or the filing
cabinet.*

Their condition differed "so markedly and uniquely
from anything [previously] reported" that Kanner
encouraged "detailed consideration of its fascinating
peculiarities."

Historical Snapshots of Modern Terminology (Physical Disabilities)

Acromegaly – A rare, progressive disease characterized by a marked enlargement of the hands, feet, and facial features—along with "changes in the body's configuration."[193] The vast majority of cases result from a benign tumor developing in the pituitary gland which, in turn, prompts an increase in the production of growth hormone (GH).[194] French neurologist Pierre Marie established *acromegaly* as a distinct clinical diagnosis in 1886 after examining two older female patients at the Salpêtrière Hospital in Paris who displayed "an enormous hypertrophy [excessive growth] of the hands and feet."[195] Subjective symptoms included headaches, visual disturbances, and an insatiable thirst. In describing one of these patients, Dr. Marie wrote:

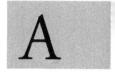

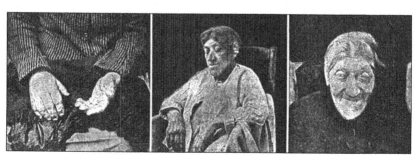

Photographs from Dr. Marie's 1885 study on Two Cases of Acromegaly.

It was at the age of twenty-four, at the time the menstruation suddenly ceased, that she noticed the sudden increase in her hands. Her face at this time also underwent changes . . . so that when the patient returned home none of her relatives could recognize her . . .. The whole feet are large, including the toes. Though the latter are increased in size, they have preserved their form, there is no true deformity; their appearance is simply that of a very big person.[196]

C **Cutaneous Geromorphism** – An abnormal skin condition that gives the appearance of very old age.[197] It was described in the late-nineteenth century by French neurologists Alexandre-Achille Souques and Jean-Martin Charcot. The condition presented itself in a young woman who arrived at the Salpêtrière Hospital at the age of twenty-one, having displayed the physical traits since childhood:

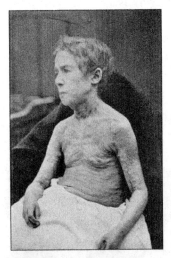

The face was most noticeably changed, and suggested a facial paralysis from the obliteration of the natural lines and lack of facial expression. The skin hung in loose folds such as are sometimes seen in extreme age, and appeared as though it had been overstretched . . . and had remained too flabby and loose in consequence.[198]

Child with "cutaneous geromorphism," photo taken at the Salpêtrière circa 1890. WELLCOME LIBRARY, LONDON.

Marfan Syndrome – A genetic disorder affecting the body's various connective tissues ("[a group of] proteins that support skin, bones, blood vessels, and other organs").[199] Symptoms can vary depending on the severity of the case; however, most people with Marfan syndrome experience problems with their circulatory and nervous systems, and display characteristic physical traits including tall height and long, thin arms and fingers. French pediatrician Bernard Marfan described the disorder in 1896, when he presented a five-year-old girl to the Medical Society of Paris. Dr. Marfan drew attention to her "disproportionately long limbs and [slender] physique," using the term *pattes d'araigness* (spider legs) to describe her appearance.[200]

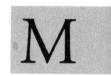

Notes

1. "Hippocrates," Microsoft® Encarta® Online Encyclopedia 2009. http://encarta.msn.com; © 1997–2009 Microsoft Corporation: All Rights Reserved.

2. Bernard Mackler, *Philippe Pinel: Unchainer of the Insane* (New York: Franklin Watts, Inc., 1968), 27.

3. Jacalyn Duffin, *History of Medicine: A Scandalously Short Introduction* (University of Toronto Press, 2010), 318.

4. This phrase appeared in: Luther V. Bell, "On a New Form of Disease," *The American Journal of Insanity*, vol. 4 (Utica: 1849–50), 99.

5. Richard H. Hutchings, *A Psychiatric Word Book: A Lexicon of Terms Employed in Psychiatry and Psychoanalysis*, 7th ed. (Utica, New York: State Hospitals Press, 1943), 16.

6. Daniel H. Tuke, ed., *A Dictionary of Psychological Medicine*, vol. 1 (Philadelphia: P. Blakiston, Son & Co., 1892), 56.

7. *Ibid*, 60.

8. *Ibid*, 61.

9. Edward Charles Spitzka, *Insanity: Its Classification, Diagnosis, and Treatment* (New York: E.B. Treat, 1889), 251.

10. Henry Johns Berkley, *A Treatise on Mental Diseases* (Ayer Publishing, 1980), 247–252.

11. Benjamin Rush, *Medical Inquiries and Observations, upon the Diseases of the Mind* (Philadelphia: 1812), 136–138.

12. Benjamin Rush, *An Inquiry into the Influence of Physical Causes upon the Moral Faculty*, Delivered Feb. 27, 1786 (Philadelphia: Haswell, Barrington, and Haswell, 1839), 1; Dr. Rush identified the moral faculty as "[the] capacity in the human mind of distinguishing and choosing good and evil, or, in other words, virtue and vice."

13. Jan Verplaetse, *Localizing the Moral Sense: Neuroscience and the Search for the Cerebral Seat of Morality* (Springer, 2009), 192–3.

14. The image is from: William Hogarth, *A Rake's Progress* (London, England: 1735).

15. Richard Noll, *The Encyclopedia of Schizophrenia and Other Psychotic Disorders* (Infobase Publishing, 2009), 51.

16. Luther V. Bell, "On a New Form of Disease," *The American Journal of Insanity*, vol. 4 (Utica: 1849–50), 97–127.

17. *Ibid*, 106–7.

18. *Ibid*, 98.

19. *Ibid*, 97.

20. Silas Durkee, *A Treatise on Gonorrhea and Syphilis* (J. P. Jewett, 1859), 110–111.

21. Leland Hinsie & Robert J. Campbell, *Psychiatric Dictionary*, 4th ed. (New York: Oxford University Press, 1970), 117.

22. *A Reference Handbook of the Medical Sciences*, vol. 5, ed. Albert H. Buck (William Wood and Company, 1902), 132.

23. Charles L. Dana, *Textbook of Nervous Diseases and Psychiatry*, sixth edition (Wm. Wood Company, 1904), 629.

24. *Borderline Personality Disorder: Clinical and Empirical Perspectives*, ed. John Clarkin et al (Guilford Press, 1991), 7.

25. Richard Noll, *The Encyclopedia of Schizophrenia and Other Psychotic Disorders* (Infobase Publishing, 2009), 125.

26.   Emil Kraepelin, *Dementia Praecox and Paraphrenia*, trans. R. Mary Barclay (Chicago Medical Book Co., 1916), 3.

27.   Robert Gibson, "Dementia Infantilis: Report of a Case," *Canadian Medical Association Journal*, vol. 80, no. 2, (January 15, 1959), 114–116.

28.   Richard H. Hutchings, *A Psychiatric Word Book*, 68.

29.   Jean-Etienne Dominique Esquirol, *Mental Maladies: A Treatise on Insanity*, trans. Ebenezer Kingsbury Hunt (Philadelphia, Lea and Blanchard, 1845), 242.

30.   *Ibid.*

31.   John G. Howells and M. Livia Osborn, *A Reference Companion to the History of Abnormal Psychology* vol. 1 (Greenwood Press, 1984), 243.

32.   Richard Noll, *The Encyclopedia of Schizophrenia and Other Psychotic Disorders* (Infobase Publishing, 2009), 130.

33.   Eugen Bleuler, *Textbook of Psychiatry*, trans. A. A. Brill (New York: The Macmillan Company, 1934), 384.

34.   http://medical-dictionary.thefreedictionary.com/dereistic+thinking

35.   Charles McCreery, *Dreams and Psychosis: A New Look at an Old Hypothesis* (Oxford Forum, 2008), 5.

36.   Sarah-Jayne Blakemore, *Autism and Asperger Syndrome*, ed. Uta Frith (Cambridge University Press, 1999), 38.

37.   David Appleton Morse, *Report on Dipsomania and Drunkenness* (United Brethren Publishing House, 1873), 7–8.

38.   J. Edward Turner, *The History of the First Inebriate Asylum in the World* (New York: J. Edward Turner, 1888), 84.

39.   David Cliffe, *A Companion to Evelyn Waugh's "Sword of Honour"* (Published online, November 8, 2001), Ch. 3, p. 1.

40.   Leland Hinsie and Robert J. Campbell, *Psychiatric Dictionary*, 4th ed. (New York: Oxford University Press, 1970), 315.

41. Theodore Millon, *Masters of the Mind: Exploring the Story of Mental Illness* (John Wiley & Sons, 2004), 176.

42. Richard H. Hutchings, *A Psychiatric Word Book*, 105.

43. Floyd M. Crandall, "Hospitalism," *Archives of Pediatrics* vol. 14, no. 6 (June, 1897), 448–454; accessed from: http://www.neonatology.org/classics/crandall.html

44. René A. Spitz, *Psychogenic Disease in Infancy*, 1952 (Prelinger Archives); This video can be viewed here: http://archive.org/details/PsychogenicD

45. Charles L. Dana, *Textbook of Nervous Diseases and Psychiatry*, sixth edition (Wm. Wood Company, 1904), 629.

46. Richard H. Hutchings, *A Psychiatric Word Book*, 127.

47. Jules Cashford, *The Moon: Myth and Image* (Basic Books, 2003), 282.

48. For instance, Dr. Jean-Étienne Dominique Esquirol believed that the high prevalence of insanity during full moons arose from the increased amount of light present (which produced "an agitating effect on all insane persons"). – John S. Stock, *A Practical Treatise on the Law of Non Compotes Mentis, or Persons of Unsound Mind* (J.S. Littell, 1839), 5.

49. Daniel Clark, "Popular Delusions about the Insane," *Appendix to the Thirty-Third Annual Report of the Inspector of Prisons and Public Charities upon the Lunatic and Idiot Asylums of the Province of Ontario* (Toronto: 1900), 6.

50. Sidney L. Pressey and Luella C. Pressey, *Mental Abnormality and Deficiency* (New York: Macmillan Co., 1926), 166.

51. Georgi Morozov and Vladimir Romasenko, *Nervous and Psychic Diseases* (Moscow: MIR Publishers, 1968), 115.

52. Emil Kraepelin, *Manic-Depressive Insanity and Paranoia*, trans. R. Mary Barclay (Edinburgh, E. & S. Livingstone, 1921), 3.

53. *Ibid*, 3–4.

54. *Ibid*, 2.

55. Richard Krafft-Ebing, *Textbook of Insanity* (F. A. Davis, 1905), 438–439.

56. Jean Esquirol, *Mental Maladies: A Treatise on Insanity*, trans. Ebenezer Kingsbury Hunt (Philadelphia: 1845), 320.

57. M. Baillarger, "Remarks Upon Monomania," *The American Journal of Insanity*, vol. IV (Utica, New York: 1847–8), 16–26.

58. Jean Esquirol, *Mental Maladies: A Treatise on Insanity*, trans. Ebenezer Kingsbury Hunt (Philadelphia: 1845), 320.

59. Amariah Brigham, "Millerism," *The American Journal of Insanity* vol. I (Utica, New York: 1844–45), 249.

60. Jean Esquirol, *Mental Maladies: A Treatise on Insanity*, trans. Ebenezer Kingsbury Hunt (Philadelphia: 1845), 331.

61. *Ibid*, 332.

62. Amariah Brigham, "Millerism," *The American Journal of Insanity* vol. I (Utica, New York: 1844–45), 252.

63. Aldous Huxley, "Madness, Badness, Sadness," *Esquire* (June 1956); quoted in *Collected Essays* (New York: Harper, 1959).

64. Bernard Mackler, *Philippe Pinel: Unchainer of the Insane* (New York: Franklin Watts, Inc., 1968), 72–73.

65. Scipion Pinel, "The Bicêtre in 1792," quoted in William and Robert Chambers, *Chambers's Edinburgh Journal*, vol. 11, no. 272 (March, 1849), 169–171.

66. Albert Deutsch, *The Mentally Ill in America: A History of their Care and Treatment from Colonial Times*, 3rd ed. (New York: Columbia University Press, 1946), 83–85.

67. Amariah Brigham, "The Moral Treatment of Insanity," *The American Journal of Insanity*, vol. 4 (July, 1847), 1.

68. Francis Tiffany, *Life of Dorothea Lynde Dix* (Boston: Houghton, Mifflin, and Company, 1890), 94.

69. Jan E. Goldstein, *Console and Classify: The French Psychiatric Profession in the Nineteenth Century* (University of Chicago Press, 2002), 146.

70. *Handbook of Psychology, vol. 1: History of Psychology*, eds. Freedheim & Weiner (John Wiley & Sons, 2003), 340.

71. Edward M. Brown, "French Psychiatry's Initial Reception of Bayle's Discovery of General Paresis of the Insane," *Bulletin of the History of Medicine*, vol. 68 (1994), 235–253.

72. Edward Charles Spitzka, *Insanity: Its Classification, Diagnosis and Treatment* (Bermingham & Co., 1883), 267.

73. James MacDonald, "Puerperal Insanity," *The American Journal of Insanity*, vol. 4 (Utica, New York: 1847–8), 113.

74. Andrea Tone, *The Age of Anxiety: A History of America's Turbulent Affair with Tranquilizers* (Basic Books, 2008), 5–6.

75. Jean Esquirol, *Mental Maladies: A Treatise on Insanity*, trans. Ebenezer Kingsbury Hunt (Philadelphia: 1845), 446.

76. Edward Seguin, *Traitement Moral, Hygiène et Éducation des Idiots* (Paris: J.B. Baillière, 1846); translated in: James W. Trent, Jr., *Inventing the Feeble Mind* (University of California Press, 1994), 45–46.

77. *The British and Foreign Medical Review*, vol. XXIV, July 1847, ed. John Forbes (London: John Churchill, 1847), 3.

78. Bernard Sachs, "On Arrested Cerebral Development, with Special Reference to its Cortical Pathology," *The Journal of Nervous and Mental Disorders*, vol. 14 (1887): 541. Bernard Sachs, "A Family Form of Idiocy, Generally Fatal, Associated with early Blindness (Amaurotic Family Idiocy)" *The Journal of Nervous and Mental Diseases*, vol. 21 (1896): 475–479.

79. Julius Parker Sedgwick, *Text-book of Pediatrics* (Philadelphia: J. B. Lippincott Company, 1922), 523.

80. William Cullen, *First Lines of the Practice of Physic*; quoted in German Berrios, *The History of Mental Symptoms: Descriptive Psychopathology since the Nineteenth Century* (Cambridge University Press, 1996), 159.

81. *The London Encyclopedia: Or Universal Dictionary of Science, Art, Literature, and Practical Mechanics*, vol. 1, ed. Thomas Curtis (London, 1829), 743.

82. Bartholomew Parr, *The London medical dictionary*, vol. 1 (T. Davison, 1809), 92, 130.

83. James Herbert McKee, *Practical Pediatrics* vol. 2 (P. Blakiston's Son, 1914), 640.

84. Sidney L. Pressey and Luella Cole Pressey, *Mental Abnormality and Deficiency* (New York: Macmillan Co., 1926).

85. *Ibid.*

86. Gilman Goodman, *The Biological Basis of Therapeutics*, 4th ed., (London: MacMillan, 1970), 121–122; The anticonvulsant properties of potassium bromide were first noted by Sir Charles Locock at a meeting of the Royal Medical and Chirurgical Society in 1857.

87. William Pryor Letchworth, *Care and Treatment of Epileptics* (New York: G. P. Putnam's Sons, 1900), 118.

88. *Ibid*, 118.

89. Richard H. Hutchings, *A Psychiatric Word Book*, 63.

90. Linus P. Brockett, "Cretins and Idiots," *The Atlantic Monthly* (February 1858).

91. Linus P. Brockett, "Idiots and the Efforts for Their Improvement," *Barnard's American Journal of Education*, vol. 1, No. 4, (Hartford, Connecticut: Case, Tiffany & Co, 1856), 40.

92. Article 31B, Section 5, *Annotated Code of the Public General Laws of Maryland*, 1951, 1977, 1989; quoted in Marilyn D. McShane and Frank P. Williams III, eds., *Encyclopedia of American Prisons* (Taylor & Francis, 1996), 558.

93. Milton Harrington, "The Problem of the Defective Delinquent," *Mental Hygiene*, vol. XIX, no. 3 (July 1935), 430.

94. Louis N. Robinson, "Institutions for Defective Delinquents," *Journal of Criminal Law and Criminology*, vol. 24, no. 2 (July–August, 1933), 353.

95. Amram Scheinfeld, *The Human Heredity Handbook* (Philadelphia: J. P. Lippincott Company, 1956), 137.

96. Peter L. Tyor and Leland V. Bell, *Caring for the Retarded in America: A History* (Greenwood Press, 1984), 6–7.

97. Charles Dickens, "Idiots," *Household Words*, June 4, 1853; www.lang. nagoya-u.ac.jp/~matsuoka/CD-Idiots.html

98. Peter L. Tyor and Leland V. Bell, *Caring for the Retarded in America: A History* (Greenwood Press, 1984), 6–7.

99. Martin W. Barr and E. F. Maloney, *Types of Mental Defectives* (Philadelphia: P. Blakiston's Son & Co., 1920), 124.

100. John Langdon Down, *On Some of the Mental Affections of Childhood and Youth* (London, J&A Churchill, 1887), 99.

101. Annesley Kenealy, "A Mad Genius: The Master Craftsman of Earlswood Asylum," *Pearson's Magazine* (1898), 98–103.

102. Geneva Handy Southall, *Blind Tom, the Black Pianist-Composer: Continually Enslaved* (Scarecrow Press, 2002), 6.

103. Martin W. Barr and E. F. Maloney, *Types of Mental Defectives* (Philadelphia: P. Blakiston's Son & Co., 1920), 18.

104. McKinney's Consolidated Laws of New York, Annotated; Book 34-A: Mental Deficiency Law, Supplement, 1926, p. 2 (New York: Edward Thompson Company, 1919).

105. John Langdon Down, "Ethnic Classification of Idiots" (1866); quoted in Peter and Greta Beighton, *The Man Behind the Syndrome* (Springer-Verlag Berlin Heidelberg, 1986), 41.

106. Alexandra Stern, *Telling Genes: The Story of Genetic Counseling in America* (JHU Press, 2012), 160.

107. Isaac Kerlin, "The Moral Imbecile," *Proceedings of the National Conference of Charities and Corrections*, vol. XVII (George H. Ellis, 1890), 244–250.

108. Thomas Lathrop Stedman, *A Practical Medical Dictionary*, 7th ed. (William Wood and Company, 1922), 627.

109. Henry H. Goddard, "Who Is a Moron?" *The Scientific Monthly*, vol. XXIV, issue 1, (1927), 41–46.

110. J. David Smith, *Minds Made Feeble: The Myth and Legacy of the Kallikaks* (Maryland: Aspen Systems Corp., 1985), 11.

111. Ebenezer Cobham Brewer, *Dictionary of Phrase and Fable* (London: Cassell and Company, 1893), 879.

112. Richard H. Hutchings, *A Psychiatric Word Book*, 168.

113. Lisa Cartwright, *Screening the Body: Tracing Medicine's Visual Culture* (University of Minnesota Press, 1995), 61.

114. *Ibid*, 62.

115. Samuel Gridley Howe, *Report Made to the Legislature of Massachusetts, upon Idiocy* (Boston: 1848), 73.

116. *Ibid*, 25.

117. Charles Bernstein, *Ninth Annual Report of the Rome Custodial Asylum*, 1903); quoted in James G. Riggs, *Hello Doctor: A Brief Biography of Charles Bernstein, M.D.* (East Aurora, New York: Roycroft Shops, 1936), 19.

118. Ebenezer Cobham Brewer, *Dictionary of Phrase and Fable* (London: Cassell and Company, 1893), 146.

119. Shaheda N. Azher and Joseph Jankovic, "Camptocormia: Pathogenesis, Classification, and Response to Therapy," *Neurology*, vol. 65 (2005), 355–359.

120. George W. Hall, "Camptocormia (Bent Back)," *The Journal of the American Medical Association*, vol. 72 (HighWire Press, 1919), 547.

121. John G. Howells and M. Livia Osborn, *A Reference Companion to the History of Abnormal Psychology* (Greenwood Press, 1984), 154.

122. Shaheda N. Azher and Joseph Jankovic, "Camptocormia: Pathogenesis, Classification, and Response to Therapy," *Neurology*, vol. 65 (2005), 355–359.

123. M. Clanet, "Jean-Martin Charcot (1825-1893)," *The International Multiple Sclerosis Journal*, vol. 15 (2008), 59–61.

124. Richard H. Hutchings, *A Psychiatric Word Book*, 154.

125. Robert Bogdan, *Freak Show: Presenting Human Oddities for Amusement and Profit* (Uni. of Chicago Press, 1990).

126. *Ibid.*

127. Richard H. Hutchings, *A Psychiatric Word Book*, 109.

128. Margaret Bancroft, "Classification of the Mentally Deficient," *Proceedings of the National Conference of Charities and Correction*, ed. Isabel C. Barrows (Boston, Massachusetts: George H. Ellis, 1901), 191–200.

129. Nicolas Andry, *Orthopaedia: Or the Art of Correcting and Preventing Deformities in Children* (London, 1743); quoted in Leonard F. Peltier, *Orthopedics: A History and Iconography* (Norman Publishing, 1993), 21.

130. Richard H. Hutchings, *A Psychiatric Word Book*, 176.

131. Elan D. Louis, "Paralysis Agitans in the Nineteenth Century," quoted in Stewart Factor and William Weiner, *Parkinson's Disease: Diagnosis & Clinical Management*, 2nd ed. (Demos Medical Publishing, 2007).

132. James Parkinson, *An Essay on the Shaking Palsy* (London: Whittingham and Rowland, 1817).

133. *Ibid*, 2, 8.

134. Edward J. Huth and T. Jock Murray, eds., *Medicine in Quotations: Views of Health and Disease Through the Ages* (Philadelphia: American College of Physicians, 2006), 283.

135. *A Dictionary of Psychological Medicine*, vol. 1, ed. Daniel H. Tuke (Philadelphia: P. Blakiston, Son & Co., 1892), 937.

136. Ebenezer Cobham Brewer, *Dictionary of Phrase and Fable* (London: Cassell and Company, 1893), 1229.

137. John Todd, "The Syndrome of Alice in Wonderland," *Canadian Medical Association Journal*, vol. 73, no. 9 (November 1, 1955), 701–2; Dr. Todd explained: "The . . . illusions of bodily distortion experienced by patients with the syndrome are comparable to the visual illusions produced by the parabolic mirrors of a fun-fair."

138. *Ibid*, 703.

139. Richard H. Hutchings, *A Psychiatric Word Book*, 35.

140. Robert M. Levy and Leonard S. Rubenstein, *The Rights of People with Mental Disabilities* (ACLU, 1996), 17.

141. Sheila Rothman, *The Discovery of the Asylum: Social Order and Disorder in the New Republic* (1971), 130.

142. *A Dictionary of Psychological Medicine*, vol. 1, ed. Daniel H. Tuke, (Philadelphia: P. Blakiston, Son & Co., 1892), 397.

143. Ebenezer Cobham Brewer, *Dictionary of Phrase and Fable* (London: Cassell and Company, 1893), 374.

144. http://en.wikipedia.org/wiki/Duns_Scotus

145. Stormy J. Chamberlain and Marc Lalande, "Angelman Syndrome, a Genomic Imprinting Disorder of the Brain," *The Journal of Neuroscience*, vol. 30, no. 30 (July 28, 2010), 9958–9963; quote on p. 9958.

146. "History of the Diagnosis," http://www.angelmanproject.com/history. htm (GeneticaLens, 2003).

147. Leland Hinsie & Robert J. Campbell, *Psychiatric Dictionary*, 4th ed. (New York: Oxford University Press, 1970), 455.

148. Lightner Witmer, *The Psychological Clinic: A Journal of Orthogenics*, vol. IV, no. 5, October 15, 1910 (Philadelphia: Psychological Clinic Press, 1910), ii.

149. *Ibid*, 554.

150. Richard H. Hutchings, *A Psychiatric Word Book*, 197.

151. *Ibid*, 201.

152. *Ibid*, 227.

153. William W. Gull, "Anorexia Nervosa," *Transactions of the Clinical Society of London*, vol. 7 (1874), 22–28.

154. Richard Noll, *The Encyclopedia of Schizophrenia and Other Psychotic Disorders* (Infobase Publishing, 2009), 53–4.

155. August Hoch, *Benign Stupors: A Study of a New Manic-Depressive Reaction Type* (Macmillan Co., 1921), 206–207.

156. Max Fink and Michael Alan Taylor, *Catatonia: A Clinician's Guide to Diagnosis and Treatment* (Cambridge University Press, 2003), 3–5.

157. M. P. Barnes, M. Saunders, T. J. Walls, I. Saunders, and C. A. Kirk, "The Syndrome of Karl Ludwig Kahlbaum" *Journal of Neurology, Neurosurgery, and Psychiatry*, vol. 49 (1986), 991–996.

158. Thomas Sutton, *Tracts on Delirium Tremens* (London: James Moyes, 1813).

159. A.D.A.M Medical Encyclopedia; accessed from: http://www.ncbi.nlm. nih.gov/pubmedhealth/PMH0001771.

160. James Conquest Cross, Prize Dissertation (for 1831), on Delirium Tremens; *Transactions of the New York State Medical Society*, Vol. 1; quoted in *The Western Journal of the Mental and Physical Sciences*, ed. Daniel Drake, M.D., Vol. VIII (Cincinnati, Ohio, 1835), 43–62; quote from page 46.

161. Einar Brünniche, "Memory images of acute, alcoholic delirium," *Bibliotek for Læger* vol. 111 (1911), 199–214.

162. Richard H. Hutchings, *A Psychiatric Word Book*, 67.

163. Georgi Morozov and Vladimir Romasenko, *Nervous and Psychic Diseases* (Moscow: MIR Publishers, 1968), 120–21.

164. Linda C. Lu and Juergen H. Bludau, *Alzheimer's Disease: Biographies of disease* (ABC-CLIO, 2011), 2.

165. Estimates courtesy of the Alzheimer's Association®; http://www.alz.org/dementia/types-of-dementia.asp

166. Alois Alzheimer, "A Characteristic Serious Disease of the Cerebral Cortex" (1907); quoted in Konrad Maurer, Stephan Volk, Hector Gerbaldo, "Auguste D and Alzheimer's disease," *The Lancet*, vol. 349 (May 24, 1997), 1548.

167. Owsei Temkin, *The Falling Sickness: A History of Epilepsy from the Greeks to the Beginnings of Modern Neurology* (JHU Press, 1994), 220–223.

168. James Donnegan, *A New Greek and English Lexicon* (Taylor, 1842), 637

169. Sydney Brooks, "A New York 'Colony of Mercy,'" *The American Monthly Review of Reviews: An International Magazine*, vol. XXI, January–June, 1900, ed. Albert Shaw (New York: The Review of Reviews Company, 1900), 313.

170. William P. Spratling, "Address," *Proceedings of the Livingston County Historical Society*, Twenty-Fifth Annual Meeting, August 21, 1899 (Geneseo, New York: Livingston Republican, 1900), 19.

171. William Pryor Letchworth, *The Care and Treatment of Epileptics* (New York: G. P. Putnam's Sons, 1900), 116.

172. *Ibid.*

173. F. A. Whitlock, *Oxford Companion to the Mind: Sir Thomas Sydenham* (Oxford University Press, 1987).

174. This belief persisted despite the fact that, as early as the mid 1600s, English physician Thomas Sydenham demonstrated the presence of hysteria in males.

175. Asti Hustvedt, *Medical Muses: Hysteria in Nineteenth-Century Paris* (W. W. Norton & Company, 2011), 19.

176. *Ibid*, 3.

177. Richard H. Hutchings, *A Psychiatric Word Book*, 122.

178. Jean-Etienne Dominique Esquirol, *Mental Maladies: A Treatise on Insanity*, trans. Ebenezer Kingsbury Hunt (Philadelphia, Lea and Blanchard, 1845), 21.

179. *Ibid.*

180. Eugen Bleuler, *Textbook of Psychiatry*, trans. A. A. Brill (New York: The Macmillan Company, 1934), 472.

181. *Ibid.*

182. Michael A. Taylor & Max Fink, *Melancholia: The Diagnosis, Pathophysiology and Treatment of Depressive Illness* (Cambridge University Press, 2006), 45–46.

183. Eugen Bleuler, *Textbook of Psychiatry*, trans. A. A. Brill (New York: The Macmillan Company, 1934), 373; Dr. Bleuler wrote: "[schizophrenia] may come to a standstill at every stage and many of its symptoms may clear up very much or altogether; but if it progresses, it leads to a dementia of a definite character."

184. *The American Journal of Psychiatry*, vol. 120 (Johns Hopkins Press, 1964), 351.

185. Eugen Bleuler, *Textbook of Psychiatry*, trans. A. A. Brill (New York: The Macmillan Company, 1934), 373.

186. Hans Asperger, "'Autistic Psychopathy' in Childhood," quoted in: *Autism and Asperger Syndrome*, ed. Uta Frith (Cambridge University Press, 1991), 37.

187. *Ibid*, 40 Image obtained from: http://kolahun.typepad.com/kolahun/2012/02/has-asperger-md-1906-1980.html

188. Alexander Crichton, *An Inquiry into the Nature and Origin of Mental Derangement: Comprehending a Concise System of the Physiology and Pathology of the Human Mind. And a History of the Passions and Their Effects*, vol. 1 (T. Cadell, Junior, and W. Davies, 1798), 272.

189. George Frederic Still, "The Ghoulstonian Lectures on Some Abnormal Psychical Conditions in Children," *The Lancet*, vol. 1 (1902), 1008–12.

190. *Autism and Asperger Syndrome*, ed. Uta Frith (Cambridge University Press, 1991), 2.

191. Leo Kanner, "Autistic Disturbances of Affective Contact," *Nervous Child* vol. 2 (1943): 217–250.

192. *Ibid.*

193. Richard H. Hutchings, *A Psychiatric Word Book*, 16.

194. Mary Lee Vance, "Acromegaly: A Fascinating Pituitary Disorder," *Neurosurgical Focus*, vol. 29, no. 4 (Oct. 2010).

195. Pierre Marie and Jose de Souza-Leite, *Essays on Acromegaly* (London: The New Sydenham Society, 1891), 18.

196. *Ibid*, 18–19.

197. Picture: Pierre-Émile Launois, *Nouvelle iconographie de la Salpêtrière clinique des Maladies du systeme nerveux* (Veuve Bebe et Cie, Libraires-Editeurs: Paris, 1891), Table IV (4) Plate XXI (21).

198. *Medical Record* vol. 40, ed. George F. Shrady (New York: William Wood and Company, 1891), 305.

199. Information from the National Institute of Arthritis and Musculoskeletal and Skin Diseases; http://www.nlm.nih.gov/medlineplus/ marfansyndrome.html

200. Peter and Greta Beighton, *The Man Behind the Syndrome* (Springer-Verlag Berlin Heidelberg, 1986), 107.

Illustration and Image Credits

Unless otherwise stated, illustrations and images in this publication are courtesy of the Museum of disABILITY History.

Chapter 1
2: Courtesy of the National Library of Medicine.
5: Courtesy of the British Museum.
9: Courtesy of the Wellcome Library, London.
13: Courtesy of the International Kraepelin Society.
16: *Right image:* Courtesy of the National Library of Medicine.
17: Courtesy of the National Library of Medicine.
22: Courtesy of the National Library of Medicine.

Chapter 2
24: Courtesy of the National Library of Medicine.
26: Courtesy of the HathiTrust Digital Library.
52: Courtesy of the National Library of Medicine.

Historical Snapshots of Modern Terminology
57: Courtesy of the Wellcome Library, London.
59: Courtesy of the Medical Museion in Copenhagen, Denmark.
64: *Top image:* Courtesy of the Wellcome Library, London.
72: Courtesy of the Wellcome Library, London.

Index